DEFEATING
DEMENTIA

DEFEATING DEMENTIA

What You Can Do to Prevent Alzheimer's and Other Forms of Dementia

RICHARD FURMAN, MD, FACS

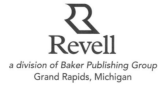

Revell

a division of Baker Publishing Group
Grand Rapids, Michigan

Published by Revell
a division of Baker Publishing Group
PO Box 6287, Grand Rapids, MI 49516-6287
www.revellbooks.com

Printed in the United States of America

Library of Congress Cataloging-in-Publication Control Number: 2017043037

The author is represented by the literary agency of Wolgemuth & Associates, Inc.

Names, details, etc. have been altered to protect the privacy of individuals.

All the proceeds will go to Samaritan's Purse for World Medical Mission.

Portions of this book have been taken from *Prescription for Life*, published by Revell, 2014.

This publication is intended to provide helpful and informative material on the subjects addressed. Readers should consult their personal health professionals before adopting any of the suggestions in this book or drawing inferences from it. The author and publisher expressly disclaim responsibility for any adverse effects arising from the use or application of the information contained in this book.

18 19 20 21 22 23 24   7 6 5 4 3 2 1

In keeping with biblical principles of creation stewardship, Baker Publishing Group advocates the responsible use of our natural resources. As a member of the Green Press Initiative, our company uses recycled paper when possible. The text paper of this book is composed in part of post-consumer waste.

To Katy and all the caregivers
who gave such loving care to Mrs. Dell

Grow old along with me—
the best is yet to be.

Robert Browning

Contents

Foreword

When I was serving as the US Senate majority leader, I regularly traveled with my close friend Dr. Furman on medical missions throughout the world. From responding to medical emergencies such as Hurricane Katrina here at home, to earthquakes in Haiti, to leading medical emergency responses more than a dozen times throughout Africa, we have operated as surgeons side by side. I know him well. He is a man of action. I have witnessed his compassion and his skills as a caregiver operating one-on-one, improving the health of the individual. He now operates in the even larger arena of interpreting the medical literature on prevention for the benefit of us all. His focus today, as so well demonstrated in *Defeating Dementia*, is to prevent health problems.

As a surgeon, you can touch hundreds, maybe thousands—but through the dissemination of medical research and public education that can shift behavior you can reach millions. We often hear the phrase "an ounce of prevention is worth a pound of cure." When it comes to health that is doubly true, because medical services account for just 10 to 15 percent of our health outcomes. The biggest determinant of health (40 percent) is human behavior: how we eat, live, work, worship, and play. The long-term success of my heart and lung transplant patients—once we get over the initial hurdle of organ rejection—is largely determined by diet, exercise, tobacco use, and related lifestyle choices.

Most Americans are familiar with actions that can be taken to reduce our risk for heart attack, stroke, cancer, diabetes, and a number of other leading ailments. But what about for Alzheimer's disease and related dementias? Every one of us is affected today in some way by Alzheimer's dementia, though clearly some much more directly than others. Current trends suggest those connections will grow closer and more painfully personal with the passing of each year. So it makes sense to learn everything we can and take control through action grounded in current medical science to alter the trajectory of those trends. It is our nation's sixth leading cause of death, yet few can answer the question, What can be done to prevent cognitive decline?

Within these covers, Dr. Furman tackles this question head-on. He shares what he has gleaned from exhaustively reviewing recent medical literature and presents what changes we can make to lessen our odds of developing Alzheimer's, as well as steps to slow the process if it has already begun. The many medical advances in recent years concerning Alzheimer's dementia, due to the use of MRI and PET brain studies, shed light on disease development and progression, as beta-amyloid protein accumulates in the brain and kills off cells well before symptoms are apparent. Dr. Furman succinctly translates these brain imaging studies to give readers a profound glimpse of the obscure happenings inside as we watch the obvious outside. Drawing upon his own enlightening observations of his mother-in-law going through the progressive stages of Alzheimer's over a fifteen-year period, he writes this compelling treatise to raise our awareness of what we can do at whatever age to counter this devastating process. While many books have been written about individuals with Alzheimer's, none has so seamlessly connected the disease biology, the patient experience, and the preventative science as Dr. Furman does so skillfully.

I first read this work, as you will, through the eyes of my own experiences. As a heart specialist and transplant surgeon, I learned what Alzheimer's does to the brain, beginning slowly but progressing day by day. In my specialty, it is broadly known that when the arteries that feed the heart become clogged with plaque, the heart muscle begins to progressively fail. Dr. Furman explains the parallel relationship that few others address: the vital connection between the health of the arteries feeding the brain and its normal functioning. Most importantly, he spells out what we can do—the specific, controllable lifestyle steps we can take to improve the supply of nutrients to the brain.

As I think back to our mission trips overseas, it was clear to Dr. Furman and me the overwhelming public health benefit we as Americans enjoy because of prevention. Childhood vaccination efforts have eradicated diseases such as smallpox, measles, and polio. Clean water and sound sanitation systems prevent waterborne illnesses and diarrhea that can be deadly to young children. Safe roads, seat belts, and airbags significantly reduce morbidity and mortality in traffic accidents, and the list goes on. Our approach to cognitive health should be no different. With over five million Americans currently living with Alzheimer's, and triple that number projected for 2050, it's time for us to consider how to be proactive in addressing this very real threat to public health. With no cure or medication yet developed to halt the progress of this debilitating disease, we must seriously consider lifestyle changes as a first line of defense.

Dr. Doug Brown, director of research and development at the Alzheimer's Society, said, "Though it's not inevitable, dementia is currently set to be the 21st century's biggest killer. We all need to be aware of the risks and start making positive lifestyle changes." And this is what Dr. Furman's book is all about: taking peer-reviewed academic research and turning it into a way of living that will support brain health.

Dr. Furman's work will serve as the definitive guide on preventative measures to decrease one's chances of developing Alzheimer's dementia. It gives specific steps to take in your everyday life to reduce risk and delay symptoms. By reading this book, you are proactively learning how to protect and preserve your brain health and longevity. I strongly encourage readers to develop the lifestyles explained in *Defeating Dementia* to help guard against one of the most dreaded diseases we know.

Senator Bill Frist

Foreword

Alzheimer's is one of the most dreaded diseases of our age. It is estimated that more than 5.5 million people in the United States alone suffer from its debilitating effects. Since the vast majority of those afflicted are over sixty-five, there are tens of millions of spouses, children, and grandchildren who sadly must learn how to deal with a loved one who is slowly slipping away.

I had always thought that there was little one could do to prevent or slow the symptoms of Alzheimer's. However, in this amazing book, *Defeating Dementia*, Dr. Richard Furman explains in an easy-to-understand and detailed way that there are actually things you can be doing right now to decrease your odds of developing Alzheimer's dementia.

I have been friends with Dr. Furman for more than four decades. I have known him as an outstanding surgeon who has spent many years operating on patients whose arteries were clogged with damaging plaque, one of the known high risk contributors to the eventual development of Alzheimer's. When his mother-in-law, Mrs. Dell, contracted

Alzheimer's, he began exhaustive research into managing the risk factors of the disease, and he found that there are a number of simple preventative measures one can take to successfully fight Alzheimer's.

What I like about this book is that it is written based on a careful review of the medical literature and is explained in such a way that everyone can understand. What I especially like is that it is a great book of hope. It gives hope that you don't have to spend the latter years of your life not recognizing or knowing your children's names, not recognizing your best friends or your spouse, and eventually becoming completely dependent on someone else to care for all your needs.

This book offers more than just hope for defeating dementia—it shares the hope for life Eternal. In the epilogue, after sharing the story of Mrs. Dell's journey with Alzheimer's, Dr. Furman relates the story of Mrs. Dell's husband at a time several years before her passing. Mr. Dell realized he himself could be on his deathbed and talked about where he planned to spend eternity. The obvious reality is this: everyone is going to die. No one can defeat the grave, but everyone can have a new body, including a new mind, by accepting Jesus as their personal Savior.

This book can change the way you live. It can give you a new hope and practical steps to deal with—and even help prevent—Alzheimer's. I encourage you to not only read it as if you were reading medical literature but also study the entire material presented—especially Mr. Dell's decision in the epilogue.

Franklin Graham

Introduction

Few times in life can you look back at one specific event that made a life-changing impression on you. But that's what happened to me one day a few years ago. I was sitting on the beach in the shade under a casuarina pine tree, reading from a stack of medical literature in preparation for writing *Prescription for Life*. I was writing about the health of the arteries and what kills more than 50 percent of all Americans—heart attacks and strokes.

Even as a surgeon, I had no in-depth medical knowledge about what causes Alzheimer's. I didn't realize the complexity of the disease process. I had not read or heard discussions concerning factors that I, or anyone else, could control in order to decrease the risk of "getting" Alzheimer's. But I did realize one thing: there is no medication that can prevent the disease, much less cure it.

In the stack of medical journal articles I was reading that afternoon, a title caught my eye: "Physical Activity, Diet, and Risk of Alzheimer's Disease." I thought for a moment,

Exercise and diet. That's interesting. I was writing *Prescription for Life* to show how exercise and diet affect the risk of heart attacks and strokes. But I had not considered how those two lifestyle choices might have an effect on Alzheimer's.

I had so many other articles to read that I started to put that one aside. But the report gave specific statistics on preventing such a dreaded disease. So I read on. That article completely changed my thinking about Alzheimer's, and I hope it will change yours too.

The article that inspired me to write this book was published in the *Journal of the American Medical Association.* It reported on a study of eighteen hundred individuals, covering a period of fourteen years, who were researched for Alzheimer's dementia. Each person was studied in terms of what foods they ate, what foods they didn't eat, and how much they exercised. Here is what the researchers found.

The first topic of the study was food. At one end of the scale were the people who ate the most red meat, fried foods, and dairy, which included cheese, butter, and cream products. These are the harmful foods containing the highest amounts of harmful fat. On the other end of the scale were those who adhered to a diet rich in fruits, vegetables, high-fiber grains and cereals, nuts, fish, and olive or canola oil rather than oils from animal fats.

Researchers concluded that *those who ate the healthy diet had a 40 percent less likelihood of developing Alzheimer's dementia* than those who ate the poor diet. Remember that number.

The second topic was exercise. On one end of the scale were the sedentary people, the couch potatoes. On the opposite end were the ones who exercised the most. *Those who exercised the most had a 48 percent lower risk for Alzheimer's dementia* than those who weren't active. Remember that number too.

Now for the most exciting part of the report. The people who did both, *the people who exercised the most and ate the healthy diet, had a 67 percent lower risk of Alzheimer's.* That's the third number I want you to remember.

What I liked most about this article was the statement at the conclusion that made a bold declaration of hope regarding steps to fight Alzheimer's. The conclusion read, "In this study, both higher Mediterranean-type diet adherence and higher physical activity were independently associated with reduced risk for Alzheimer's Disease." Exercise and diet are two lifestyle choices you can make to decrease your chances of developing Alzheimer's.

I reread the article, underlining the numbers 40, 48, and 67. I couldn't help myself. I got up out of my lounge chair and started showing the article to five or six couples I knew. Every one of them was astounded. Just like me, they couldn't believe there was actually something they could be doing that could delay, defer, or even help prevent Alzheimer's.

"Just remember those three numbers," I told them. "The next time you want the bad foods or to sit idle all day, just recall 40, 48, and 67. Food, exercise, both. 40, 48, 67."

The next morning I knew I had gotten my point across to at least one of them. He waved to me and said, "40, 48, 67." That's all he said. That's all he had to say.

That one article changed my thinking about Alzheimer's from that day on. I knew right then I had to go back to the medical literature and look up specific articles about what can be done to reduce the risk of Alzheimer's. What I found was almost shocking to me.

Alzheimer's is not an unknown entity that happens with no cause. It develops more often in connection with certain risk factors. The good news is that those risk factors are controllable. There are preventive steps you can take to fight the dreaded disease process of dementia.

We once accepted mental decline as "just a part of aging." But today is different. *Alzheimer's disease affects 9.7 percent of people older than seventy.* A survey of people over fifty-five revealed that Alzheimer's is feared more than any other disease. That includes heart attacks and strokes. It is even more dreaded than cancer. More people are becoming more aware of what they can do to avoid ending up as part of that 9.7 percent.

Today we're learning that we can stall or perhaps even prevent Alzheimer's dementia by making better choices about the amount of exercise we do each day, the foods we eat and the foods we avoid, and what we weigh.

That is what this book is about. It is a guideline for lifestyle changes you can make, starting today, that can make a difference in your future. It's about understanding Alzheimer's in today's world.

If you knew there were changes you could make that would reduce your chances of developing Alzheimer's, would you make them? If you tested positive for Alzheimer's, would you change your lifestyle habits? Even if you tested negative for Alzheimer's, would you change your lifestyle habits to prevent it from happening in the future? *"It is something everybody ought to know."* I read those words in a medical journal article detailing new findings about Alzheimer's. New studies reveal there is hope to markedly decrease your odds of developing the most dreaded disease in later life.

As a vascular surgeon, I spent many years operating on arteries that were filled with obstructive plaque buildup that resulted in a decrease of blood flowing to the brain. I began reading about factors that increased the odds of developing Alzheimer's. But more importantly, the medical literature also showed you could play a protective role in lessening your chance of developing the disease. I was surprised at what I found. Numerous studies utilizing brain-imaging techniques examined the progressive process of Alzheimer's dementia. Researchers found that a greater percentage of people who had certain risk factors developed Alzheimer's than did the individuals without those factors. The big takeaway was that those risk factors are *controllable. There are preventive steps you can take to fight the dreaded disease process of dementia.* I want to motivate you to begin making lifestyle changes that can lower your chances of developing Alzheimer's. You do that by lowering your odds of developing the disease process we can see in the brain-imaging studies, images that give a picture of what is happening even before the initial symptoms. There is no cure. Once Alzheimer's begins, it slowly progresses until it eventually causes death to the nerve cell it has affected. That cell will never again function. There is no pill you can take that halts the progression of what is happening. There is no known way to reverse the symptoms of what has already taken place in your brain. However, today there is hope. Controlling certain lifestyles is your only hope for prevention of Alzheimer's, as well as slowing or halting the progression once it has begun.

I believe *Defeating Dementia* will be the most informative book about Alzheimer's and other age-related dementias you will ever read. I don't say that in a prideful manner. No other book takes you through the biological process of Alzheimer's in conjunction with the day-to-day life experiences of someone who has the disease. I watched my mother-in-law, Mrs. Dell, go from being symptom-free until the inevitable finale. This book explains what is happening biologically within the brain of someone with Alzheimer's while also following a person's behavior through the life-changing process as the disease slowly progresses.

I will explain medical reports that expose certain risk factors closely associated with the development of Alzheimer's. But more importantly, this book explains what you can do to fight these factors and significantly decrease your odds of getting Alzheimer's or slow the progression if you are already having symptoms.

If you visited your physician and took a mental test for early signs of Alzheimer's, would your lifestyle habits change if you tested positive?

I bet they would. But why wait when you can start a new course today?

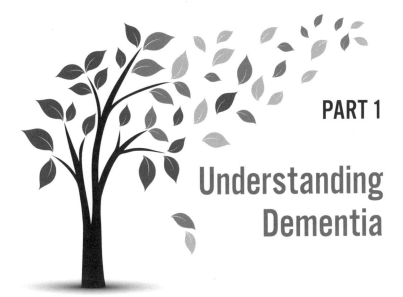

PART 1

Understanding Dementia

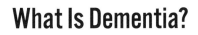

1

What Is Dementia?

Dementia Defined

If you had mentioned "dementia" to Mrs. Dell, she would not have known exactly what you were talking about. She had heard of Alzheimer's disease but didn't realize that Alzheimer's is a type of dementia.

Dementia is a condition in which the brain gradually loses its ability to think and remember clearly. It involves a decline in memory or other thinking skills—such as judgment, orientation, comprehension, and language—that affects a person's ability to carry out everyday activities. Whenever nerve cells in the brain are significantly damaged, the result is eventually dementia.

Dementia begins with damage to a number of nerve cells followed by initial symptoms beginning to show. As more nerve cells are damaged and eventually die, more symptoms occur, and the individual starts having more difficulty with memory and the ability to think clearly. Their behavior also begins to change. No one notices these symptoms at first, but as more brain cells die, the symptoms become more noticeable. Eventually, one's ability to carry out daily activities becomes so impaired that someone else has to assist them in their everyday routines. This is the point at which a person is given the diagnosis of dementia. Perhaps the person first loses the ability to drive to the store. Then they are unable to perform basic functions such as dressing themselves or walking or eating without assistance. Eventually, they become bedridden and require care around the clock. Dementia is fatal, but the sad part of dementia is that life is gone long before death arrives. An article published in the medical journal *Annals of Internal Medicine* explains the definition of dementia best. Dementia is characterized by a change in memory, plus judgment, orientation, comprehension, or language, that is severe enough to interfere with daily life. We will cover the three stages of Alzheimer's shortly and you will see that the term *dementia* corresponds with the beginning of the third stage of Alzheimer's. When a person's memory or reasoning or thought or understanding or awareness gets to the point of interfering with their daily life, from that point on, the process will be called *Alzheimer's dementia.*

One other word you will see frequently mentioned in these medical reports is the word *cognition.* That word is used in the evaluation of mental testing of Alzheimer's that relates to the participant's memory, awareness of what is going on around them, comprehension and understanding of instructions, or their reasoning in making good decisions. The tests that are given to evaluate whether the Alzheimer's is progressing or not is a measure of cognition. As your cognition worsens, so does the degree of Alzheimer's progress.

Alzheimer's Dementia

I have had people ask if a particular person had Alzheimer's or dementia. One individual told me that both his grandfather and father lost their memory and ended up bedridden and dependent on others. He said his grandfather had dementia and his father had Alzheimer's. They were different diseases in his thinking. If you say someone has Alzheimer's, most people have a picture in mind of what is going on with that individual. They have known people with Alzheimer's, have seen such people in movies, or have read books about such people. But if you were to tell the same people that someone has dementia, the picture that comes to mind is not nearly as clear. Most people are not sure what dementia is, and many think dementia and Alzheimer's are different disease processes. The fact is that Alzheimer's is a form of dementia. We will cover the three stages of Alzheimer's later, and you will see that dementia corresponds with the third stage of Alzheimer's.

Alzheimer's dementia is the most common form of dementia. Alzheimer's dementia is a complex entity. From a medical standpoint, we do not yet know what the initial step in the process is or what exactly causes Alzheimer's dementia to get worse. We do know there are two basic markers within the brains of Alzheimer's patients. These two protein products are called beta-amyloid and tau. In earlier years, to make the diagnosis, one had to perform an autopsy on someone with dementia symptoms in order to see the beta-amyloid plaques and the tau tangles imbedded in certain parts of the brain. In more recent years, brain-imaging devices have been developed that can detect the buildup of these products while a person is still alive. This process has been found to begin more than twenty years prior to any symptoms.

We also know there is more to Alzheimer's than genes. A report in the medical journal *Experimental Gerontology* stated that Alzheimer's is a chronic degeneration process in which *less than 5 percent of all cases are solely due to genetics.* If you had asked Mrs. Dell, she would have said Alzheimer's is caused by a person's genes. She would have been partially right, because a gene that is passed on in families can affect a person early on, usually between the ages of thirty and sixty. This type of Alzheimer's is called familial Alzheimer's disease. Very few people who develop Alzheimer's have this early-onset type. It accounts for less than 5 percent of overall cases.

What is more common is called sporadic Alzheimer's disease, and this usually occurs later in life, after the age of sixty. A gene called APOe4 makes a person more vulnerable to this type of Alzheimer's disease. About 20 percent of Americans have this gene, but not everyone with it will end up with Alzheimer's, and some people without the gene develop Alzheimer's. The gene doesn't cause the disease, but it can increase the risk.

The bottom line is this: you can't change your inheritance, but you can make lifestyle changes to lower your risk of developing such a dreaded disease.

It wasn't well known back in the day when Mrs. Dell was living a "normal" life, but now the Alzheimer's Association says that about *half of all people over the age of eighty-five have Alzheimer's*. If Mrs. Dell had known, perhaps she would have taken steps at a younger age to help prevent it or at least postpone the symptoms. She did not realize there were things she could do to slow or stop the progression even after she began showing symptoms.

Mrs. Dell had no idea what was happening between and within the cells of her brain. It would be twenty years before the initial symptoms would show themselves. Her life looked completely normal. She was happily married, had one married daughter, and embraced life to the fullest. Her days were fairly routine. She awoke early, fixed her husband's breakfast, then turned to her favorite hobby, the colorful, blooming flower garden completely covering the front yard.

Every afternoon Mrs. Dell drove to the grocery store to pick up what she needed for dinner. It was a small store, and she knew the owners by name. She charged everything each day and paid her invoice once a month. The one item she replenished on a daily basis was ice cream. Strawberry was her favorite. On Saturdays she would buy extra for the weekend because the store was closed on Sundays.

Every night for dessert she had her pint of ice cream. But that wasn't her only addiction. Mr. Dell brought home boxes of ice cream bars. There were six in a box, and her habit was one mid-morning and another in the middle of the afternoon.

Other than ice cream, she ate fairly normally for someone living in the South. She didn't like fish but would eat anything else—beef, pork, a lot of hamburgers, anything fried, even fried green tomatoes.

Her blood pressure was "a little high," as she liked to say with a laugh. But to her, "a little high" rather than "really high" meant that if she missed taking her blood pressure medicine now and then, it didn't make that much difference.

Mrs. Dell had no clue what beta-amyloid was nor that it was beginning to build up in her brain. Neither did she realize that Alzheimer's disease was one of the most dreaded diseases there is. That was not something anyone talked much about back then, even though Mrs. Dell's mother had died with Alzheimer's. She didn't know about certain genes that would make her more vulnerable to Alzheimer's, nor did she have any idea that certain genes would cause the disease early in life rather than late. All she knew was that her mother had developed it in her later years, and she was thankful that she had no such symptoms at her age. Mrs. Dell believed there was nothing that could be done to prevent Alzheimer's, delay its onset, or slow its progression. She accepted it as just a part of aging.

Vascular Dementia

The second most common form of dementia is caused by disease in the arteries leading to the brain and within the brain. This is called vascular dementia. The symptoms of Alzheimer's dementia and vascular dementia are practically indistinguishable, but pathological findings within the brain tissues reveal which type of problem is causing the symptoms of dementia.

If you were to do autopsy studies on the brains of people who have such symptoms, you would find certain specific abnormalities in the brain. If you were to look under a microscope at a thin slice of a particular area of the brain of someone who had the symptoms of forgetfulness or problems with their thinking process, you may see some unusual-looking protein plaques surrounding an area of brain cells that had died. If you looked closer inside those cells and saw a special type of protein called tau and saw these strands of tau protein were all tangled up, you would have the combination of findings for the diagnosis of *Alzheimer's dementia*.

As we already discussed, the brains of people with Alzheimer's dementia contain beta-amyloid plaques and tau tangles. The brains of those with vascular dementia contain very few of these plaques or tangles but do contain medium-sized or smaller arteries that became diseased and closed off from an inflammatory response with bleeding or became plugged due to plaque buildup within their walls. The autopsies of such brains would reveal large areas of brain damage as a result of a stroke. In such cases, the patients most likely experienced a stroke that was obvious to themselves and everyone else. It may have affected speech or some type of motor movement. This may have been followed sooner or later by the dementia symptoms we have been discussing. This form of vascular dementia is a result of disease of the larger arteries to the brain.

There is another form of vascular dementia that is different from the kind that reveals large strokes at autopsy. In this second form, autopsies of brain tissue reveal blockages in extremely small micro-arteries, and only a very small area of brain tissue is affected. Such areas are also the result of a stroke, but the blockage was so small and the area of brain tissue affected so petite that no symptoms of a stroke occurred. The patient didn't even know they had a light stroke. Such a stroke is called a silent stroke, and a multitude of such events can lead to vascular dementia.

This type of stroke was highlighted in an eye-opening study done by the National Alzheimer's Coordinating Center and published in the medical journal *Neurology*. In an autopsy study of brains, *researchers found that 79.6 percent of individuals showing evidence of a stroke upon examination of the brain did not have a history of a stroke during their lifetimes.* They did not have any symptoms.

If a small stroke is a little bit larger, the patient may witness a tinge of a problem that lasts only a short time, and then they completely recover. Such a stroke is called a transient ischemic attack or TIA. The symptoms are very transient, or brief, and then they disappear and the person is back to normal.

If I were back in medical school taking notes on a lecture on vascular dementia, I would write a short summary statement like this: a significant part of preventing dementia is the health of my arteries—from my largest artery to my smallest.

The Connection between Alzheimer's Dementia, Vascular Dementia, and Mixed Dementia

If you were to go to your doctor with memory problems or with difficulty making decisions or because you weren't able to figure out how to do something you used to do well, they would not be able to tell you definitively whether you had Alzheimer's or problems in your brain caused by disease of the arteries. If you presented with memory symptoms, would the cause be solely beta-amyloid plaques, solely problems with the arteries, or a combination of the two?

The answer to that question is that the majority of Alzheimer's cases have a mixed cause. Examinations of brain structure reveal a mixture of the Alzheimer's beta-amyloid plaques *and* problems with the arteries of the brain.

An article published in *Biomechanical Pharmacology* concerned Alzheimer's dementia and vascular dementia. The report stated that *Alzheimer's is a mixed disease and that the idea that these entities are completely separate has vanished.*

You might think it would be simple to figure out if dementia were caused either by those beta-amyloid plaques and tau tangles that make the diagnosis of Alzheimer's dementia or by the disease of the arteries that make the diagnosis of vascular dementia. But it is not that simple.

An article in the medical journal *Lancet* reported that the majority of dementia in the aging population is a mixture of plaques and tangles with arterial involvement. Researchers pointed out that if they examined the brains of individuals over the age of eighty who had been diagnosed with Alzheimer's, they would likely not find only plaques or only blocked arteries as the sole cause. This combination of beta-amyloid plaques and arterial disease is called mixed dementia. A Statement for Healthcare Professionals from the American Heart Association/American Stroke Association states that a mixed cause, including the arterial component and the Alzheimer's component, is the most common explanation for cognitive impairment in aging. This study showed that *the effects of arterial disease on the brain were found in 84 percent of Alzheimer's patients.*

Another statement from the medical literature concerning the intertwining of Alzheimer's dementia and vascular dementia is found in the medical journal *Archives of Neurology*. It stated, "Although Alzheimer's dementia and vascular dementia have traditionally been viewed as distinct disorders, it is now generally agreed that the two *rarely* occur in isolation." The article pointed out that what is a risk factor for one is a risk factor for the other. With there being no medication that can prevent or cure Alzheimer's, modifying your lifestyle to alleviate the risk factors remains the cornerstone for the prevention of Alzheimer's.

Several studies have found that in patients with a combination of Alzheimer's disease and arterial disease, fewer of the hallmark beta-amyloid plaques are necessary to cause dementia symptoms if there is associated arterial disease. A key reminder is that the greater the decrease in the flow of blood in the brain, the greater the decline in cognitive function. We know steps that can be taken to prevent the arterial part of the problem. *The health of your arteries is a key player that you control in the fight against Alzheimer's.*

It is not known whether arterial problems are the primary causes of Alzheimer's or whether damage to the arteries makes a person more susceptible to the formation of beta-amyloid plaques in the brain. Either way, arterial damage lowers the threshold for the symptoms of Alzheimer's disease to manifest themselves. Even though the overall cause of Alzheimer's is complex, it is important to understand as many of the causative factors as possible if your ultimate goal is prevention.

Whether you have high LDL cholesterol or are overweight or don't exercise or have high blood pressure or diabetes—you want to go after any risk factor that shows up in so many people who have Alzheimer's. You want to fight the good fight.

Mrs. Dell didn't undergo an autopsy. No slices were ever taken of her brain. I wonder what was going on inside her nerve cells. As I read the medical literature, I got a good visualization of what happens to those with dementia. As you continue to learn more about the medical aspect of the progression of Alzheimer's, you too can have the same understanding of what goes on in the brain. The more you know and understand what is going on in the brain, the better chance you have of preventing the ongoing process that leads to dementia.

For many years, I flew my own plane. Mr. Dell had told me that as far as he knew, Mrs. Dell had never flown in a plane. So I invited her to experience the excitement of flying ten thousand feet above the city to see the amazing view I knew she would enjoy. One sunny afternoon we took off and flew for what seemed like hours. At one point, we were just above the clouds. She looked out her window, then at me, and gave a big smile as she spoke so authoritatively. "I just love flying." She turned and looked back at the bank of fluffy white clouds. Her statement took me by surprise since I had been informed she had never been in a plane.

"Have you flown before?" I asked inquisitively.

"Oh, sure. It's so much fun."

"Where have you flown?" I waited expectantly to see what kind of answer she would come up with.

"Oh, I flew at the county fair when I was fourteen. They had a pilot who would fly you around the fairgrounds. You could even see the people on the Ferris wheel. My dad paid to let me go. I just loved it." I said no more.

Looking back to that day of flying, I now realize the disease was already building up within the nerve cells of her brain.

That day she was "normal." No symptoms. But now, knowing how the disease begins and progresses without anyone suspecting it has started, I realize Alzheimer's had already begun. Changes were already happening to her—long before any symptoms stuck their head out from the horrible shadows of Alzheimer's.

2

The Stages of Alzheimer's

When did Mrs. Dell initially begin developing Alzheimer's? Most people think Alzheimer's is something that starts around age sixty-five and progressively becomes worse as a person ages. Did Mrs. Dell's problem with her memory and thinking and planning begin within a few weeks?

Or months?

Or did it start twenty years earlier?

Or even thirty?

Reports and studies now reveal that the initial cellular damage in the brain begins twenty to thirty years before the first symptoms start to show. Recent advances in brain-imaging technology give us new ways to see what is going on inside a person's brain. A basic understanding of what these studies show will make it easier for you to realize there are certain factors you can control to help prevent Alzheimer's.

Stick with me. We will stay with the basics, but understanding them will help convince you that there are certain lifestyle choices you will emphatically want to embrace, as well as certain factors you will run from as fast as you can.

Could anything have been done in the twenty-plus years before Mrs. Dell had symptoms that could have prevented Alzheimer's from stealing her life? Was there anything she could have been doing earlier in life that would have significantly lowered her chances of developing Alzheimer's?

The medical literature thinks so. You can't prevent what your genes do, but there are harmful causes you can counteract by simply making some lifestyle changes. An article in the medical journal *Lancet* stated that *up to half of Alzheimer's cases can be attributed to* preventable *factors*.

Back in Mrs. Dell's younger years, I wish we had known two things. First, that Mrs. Dell had deposits of beta-amyloid plaques beginning to form in certain areas of her brain before any symptoms ever showed their faces. Second, that there were lifestyle changes she could have made that would have lowered her risk of Alzheimer's.

But we didn't know. Back then there were no brain-imaging studies that showed what was going on in her brain years before she had symptoms. Little was known about certain lifestyle changes that can reduce the risk of such symptoms. And little was known about actions that can reduce the progression of the disease after symptoms appear.

If only Mrs. Dell could have known. Perhaps she could have changed some of her lifestyle choices. But she didn't know the damage to her brain was already happening. Her doctors didn't know. Now, more and more studies show that action can be taken; many things can be done to help with prevention. More risk factors are being identified that are associated with people who have Alzheimer's. Specific brain-imaging studies now show, even prior to any symptoms, the plaques and tangles that are the hallmark of Alzheimer's. And even more important, the same brain-imaging studies reveal that certain individuals who live specific healthy lifestyles end up not having the plaques and tangles of Alzheimer's dementia.

Mrs. Dell was a beautiful, vivacious woman. She kept her blonde hair brushed and looked "picture ready" every time I saw her. Her smile met you first, as soon as your eyes met hers. She was kind and friendly to everyone. Mr. and Mrs. Dell were an amazing couple. You might see them working in the yard together, but he knew not to interfere with any of her flowers.

I remember when Mr. Dell first suspected that something wasn't quite right with his wife. I saw a glint of apprehension in his face when he spoke. Little things made him feel there was something different about the love of his life. He couldn't put his finger on anything specific, but Mrs. Dell seemed to be getting a little more forgetful.

She had lived her life with precision. She had woken up to enjoy the sunrise at 6:30 sharp for years. But now she overslept five or ten minutes. "Even until seven one morning," Mr. Dell said. What he told me was not enough to make me concerned. To me, nothing he described sounded like a stroke or brain tumor or anything serious. I encouraged him and told him we were all getting older.

Stage 1

In stage 1, even though individuals have no symptoms of Alzheimer's, they have measurable changes that can be seen with special imaging studies of the brain. Today, changes can be detected in cerebrospinal fluid taken by a needle placed through your back into the area of fluid around the spinal cord. Some changes can be detected by specific markers found in the blood of Alzheimer's individuals.

Most people will not get these studies performed on themselves, but everyone can develop a preventive lifestyle, whether there is any problem within your brain or not. You need to begin with prevention because no drug slows or stops the damage to dying brain cells in Alzheimer's disease.

Controlling your lifestyle is the only "preventive medicine" available.

The medical studies we will look at use two terms almost interchangeably. They are *cognitive decline* and *Alzheimer's*. Both are relevant to each other and interrelated. Take a minute to register the difference between *cognitive decline* and *Alzheimer's*.

Stage 1 of Alzheimer's is the period before an individual shows problems with memory or mental acuity, similar to the "normal" day I took Mrs. Dell flying. The process of Alzheimer's has started in the brain, but neither the person nor anyone else knows it because they haven't started exhibiting symptoms. There is no cognitive mental decline because enough good neurons are continuing to work in order for the person to carry out their everyday activities.

If you are over forty, the process could already have begun in your brain. There are no symptoms, and the diagnosis is called preclinical or presymptomatic Alzheimer's. This stage can begin twenty years prior to any symptoms. Some reports say even thirty.

In an Alzheimer's Association study, researchers studied 672 participants who did not have any symptoms of Alzheimer's. These individuals were studied using a special brain-imaging test that measured the thickness of different parts of the brain. As the plaques that are the hallmark of Alzheimer's begin to appear in the brain, the cells begin to die off and that area of the brain becomes thinner and less dense. The tests detected these specific changes where damage had already happened.

The conclusive finding of the study was that *even though these individuals were asymptomatic, the damaging process that leads to the symptoms of Alzheimer's was already in progress.*

An article published in the medical journal *Alzheimer's and Dementia* stated that a consensus has emerged in the

Alzheimer's research field that strategies of prevention should be initiated as early as possible before symptoms begin. The focus of prevention, therefore, has shifted to the stage 1 period. If you don't have any symptoms concerning your memory or thought processes, congratulations—now is the time to start defeating dementia.

Because a medical cure for Alzheimer's seems unlikely or even impossible, prevention aimed at the asymptomatic individual is the most powerful weapon we presently have against Alzheimer's. Symptoms usually happen after midlife, so if you are between forty and sixty years of age, this is the time to work on avoiding risk factors that can lead to Alzheimer's. The good news is that most of the risk factors related to Alzheimer's are modifiable with lifestyle changes.

Mrs. Dell had visited her friend who lived about fifteen miles out in the country many times before. She didn't have any trouble finding the house that day. But as she left to return home, the problem began. Mr. Dell explained to me what Mrs. Dell had related to him about her journey home. "She said she recalled leaving the house and driving a lot farther than she normally had to drive to get back home. She said she had other things on her mind and wasn't thinking about going straight home. She couldn't recall exactly where she went, but it took her almost two hours to get back to our house. When she told me that, it scared me a little, but she seemed completely normal after she got home."

Mr. Dell had come home from work early that day and wondered where she was. He wondered whether he should take her to the doctor to see if anything was wrong. He recently had heard about someone having high blood pressure and having some spells in which they became a little confused. Mrs. Dell was on medication for high blood pressure, but Mr. Dell thought hers was under control.

So the doctor's visit was postponed.

I asked Mr. Dell if he could think of anything else that seemed unusual.

"I've been thinking about a few little things that didn't seem too significant at the time, but now I am wondering. The first thing was when we were in the car. I was driving, and we were in heavy traffic. I asked her to turn the air conditioner on, and she looked at the dash for a minute or so and then looked back out the window. In a little bit, I asked her again to adjust the air conditioner, and she did the same thing. She just looked at the controls but didn't turn it on or adjust the fan speed or anything. I finally did it myself but wondered why she hadn't done it. I think that was the first time I thought something just wasn't right. I didn't think anything else about it. Until now." Mr. Dell paused a second, then one more example came to mind.

"Something I just thought of. Last week she was calling a good friend on the phone. I was sitting in the living room, and she was sitting on the couch. Her friend's husband answered the phone, and I heard them speaking. Then she waited for him to get his wife to the phone. It wasn't but a minute or two before she started explaining to her friend that she was going to have to call her back because she had forgotten exactly why she had called her." Mr. Dell began slowly shaking his head. "Now that I think about it, that just doesn't seem right."

I began wondering if perhaps she was having multiple light strokes called TIAs (transient ischemic attacks). People with high blood pressure can have these miniature strokes. She could have small blockages or bleeds in the arteries in her brain or even a partial blockage in a larger artery feeding the brain. I didn't mention these possibilities to Mr. Dell because I didn't want to scare him about something that might not be happening.

I asked, "Has she fallen or hit her head? Has she complained about any pain in her chest, tingling in her hands, being dizzy, or having headaches?"

"No."

"Has she been taking any supplements or any new medicines she hasn't taken before? Side effects from some supplements can cause problems."

"No, none of that, but there is one more thing that comes to mind. You know she is very methodical. Every morning she makes the bed and arranges everything neatly, making sure everything looks perfect. She even puts my shoes in a neat row in my closet. Maybe once a week now, I get home and the bed isn't made. A few times I made it up myself, but when bedtime came, she didn't mention it."

I asked Mr. Dell if he had ever thought about taking her to the doctor for any of these concerns.

"I thought about it but kept putting it off because I didn't think any of these things were bad enough to require a doctor. If something was really wrong, I thought it would either go away or eventually get worse. My plan was to take her if she got worse."

I advised him he should take Mrs. Dell to the doctor. "She needs her blood pressure checked for one thing. And she will probably undergo some tests to make sure she doesn't have anything going on with her brain."

I didn't mention the possibility of Alzheimer's, but I began thinking of where that path could lead if her symptoms turned out to be the beginning of Alzheimer's. She would require assistance, and her independence would come to an end. For the remainder of her days, she would have to depend on someone to help her. Initially, this person would probably be Mr. Dell, but the day would come when more assistance would be needed, and finally she would need constant help for every activity from eating to going to the bathroom.

I didn't want to talk to Mr. Dell about these thoughts.

"I think I would take her to her doctor," I said.

Stage 2

Stage 1 Alzheimer's disease occurs before any noticeable symptoms such as memory loss are evident to the individual or anyone else. During this time period, damage is happening, but the healthier sections of the brain are able to compensate for the ongoing injury happening in other areas.

Stage 2 is the period between the time a person begins having symptoms and they become dependent on someone else to carry out their daily routines. Stage 2 is the transitional stage between the initial symptoms and the loss of independence. In stage 2, symptoms are apparent, and now the person or someone else can recognize what is happening. Beta-amyloid plaque has built up enough in a particular portion of the brain to impair the normal function of that area. With Alzheimer's, this impairment usually involves memory.

Stage 2 is called MCI or Mild Cognitive Impairment Alzheimer's. The word *cognitive* means reasoning. Individuals experience a loss of their reasoning ability. This can include memory, rational thinking, or perception of what is going on around them.

MCI Alzheimer's is not full-blown Alzheimer's dementia in which a person is dependent on someone else to assist them in their everyday life, but it is on the road to that stage of Alzheimer's dementia. In MCI, there is a continual, progressive decline in mental acuity.

At this point, even though they remain independent, a person begins having memory problems or judgment difficulties that affect their daily life. They can't remember where they left their keys or where they put something they meant to take with them. They have trouble planning their day or experience difficulty with something they commonly do, such as writing checks and balancing their checkbook.

They get confused as to which day it is or which month. They stop in mid-sentence trying to think of a word or a place or someone's name. Activities may be more difficult to do and may take greater effort, but people in stage 2 can still do them and can get through the day on their own. Yet a report in the *European Journal of Pharmacology* pointed out that "persons with mild cognitive impairment progress to Alzheimer's disease at the rate of nearly 10% to 15% per year."

Once symptoms are present in stage 2, standard mental tests can measure how much a person's thinking process is declining. If the scores are decreasing, the person is considered to be in cognitive decline. Cognitive decline simply means the person's reasoning, rational thinking, perception, and overall intellect have declined. They don't think and reason as well as they did earlier. Of course, they don't have to take a test to determine this. Usually their spouse or friends notice a decline in how they are behaving mentally.

According to the Alzheimer's Association, as many as 10 to 20 percent of Americans who are sixty-five and older have MCI. This is why it is so important to learn all you can about slowing down the process or even preventing it from proceeding to full-blown Alzheimer's dementia. Just because someone has MCI doesn't mean they will eventually not recognize their spouse or children. There are things that can be done to help. Controlling the LDL cholesterol that is getting into your arteries that causes problems to the normal flow of blood to your brain, managing high blood pressure, getting to an ideal weight, especially if you have diabetes, and exercising are all lifestyle habits you can control that can reduce the likelihood that MCI will progress to that much-dreaded next stage of Alzheimer's dementia. The best time to develop the proper lifestyle habits to deter Alzheimer's is before symptoms appear. The next best time to commit to lifestyle changes is during stage 2. Just because the process has begun doesn't mean a person is destined to lose their independence. Just because they are becoming a little forgetful and have developed stage 2 MCI doesn't mean stage 3 is imminent.

A study published in the journal *Alzheimer's Research and Therapy* reported that 87 percent of individuals who developed MCI had at least one modifiable risk factor. That means a great majority of people with stage 2 Alzheimer's can lower their risk of the disease progressing by changing certain lifestyle factors.

An article in the *Journal of the American Medical Association* concerning stage 2 MCI Alzheimer's warned of the acceleration of the progression of Alzheimer's from the time of the initial symptoms to the time of full-blown Alzheimer's. *Several risk factors lead to this acceleration process, and these factors are controllable by how a person lives.* A person actually has some control over the speed of progression of symptoms and should do everything possible to take their foot off the accelerator of this disease. For anyone who may have even the initial symptoms, this article gives encouragement regarding how to *prevent* the progression or at least *slow down* its acceleration by combating the risk factors you will learn about later in this book. You may be wondering, what can I do? What changes should I make? Here they are in a nutshell.

Get at least thirty minutes a day of aerobic exercise that increases the workload on your heart, the organ that pumps oxygen and nutrient-rich blood to every one of those one hundred billion brain cells.

Learn which foods to eat and which to avoid. Fish will become the basic "meat" in your diet, along with olive oil and nuts. All three of these foods are healthy in the mono and polyunsaturated fats that protect the smaller arteries within as well as the larger ones leading to the brain. You will avoid the saturated fats in red meat and dairy products like cheese, cream, and butter. You will develop the habit of eating more fruits and vegetables, whole grain fiber, peas, and beans. Your eating lifestyle will develop into better eating habits. Foods you never thought you could live without will become foods you don't want. You will lose a desire to taste them because you know the role they play in harming your brain.

These lifestyle choices will become easier and easier as you remember how they impact what is going on inside your brain. If you smoke, you will think differently when you realize smokers face a 45 percent greater risk for developing dementia than someone who does not smoke. The same is true when someone who is a heavy drinker realizes that too much alcohol can have significant negative impacts on your brain.

I wish we had known these things when Mrs. Dell was diagnosed with "probable Alzheimer's." Perhaps she would have done something to change the path she was on. But we didn't know then what we know now.

At the end of stage 2, it becomes clear that the individual can't continue carrying out their daily activities without some help. Their memory problems increase, and their symptoms become more significant. There are noticeable changes in their personality and behavior. They become confused as to time or place. They forget where they are going or lose their ability to think things through. They can't operate the stove or the microwave properly. They begin to suspect that something or someone is out to get them. They can't carry on normally. They have to be helped. Yet they argue that they can carry on without help. They usually do not realize anything is wrong.

At the initial visit, the doctor examined Mrs. Dell and asked some questions. He ordered some studies and told the Dells what he was suspecting but wanted them to come back in two weeks.

Life went on fairly normally for Mrs. Dell during the two weeks prior to her follow-up appointment. She didn't seem all that concerned. But Mr. Dell related to me that they were the worst two weeks of his life. He explained what the doctor had told them at the first visit. "The doctor said it was probably Alzheimer's. He said it most likely had been developing for many years. We just hadn't realized the little things that pointed toward it." Mr. Dell paused, held up his hand, and leaned forward. "It wasn't what he said but the way he spoke.

His voice came out closer to a whisper than his normal tone, like it was some kind of secret."

Mr. Dell's face tightened as he continued explaining more of what the doctor had said. "I got to thinking about the little things he said she probably had been doing that we all thought were normal, like misplacing something. She couldn't remember where she left her coat. She left her purse at a restaurant and had to go back, or she had the waiter put leftover food in a container and then she left it on the table when we walked out. So many little things happen that you think are a part of normal aging. And they are—for some."

Mr. Dell hesitated an awkwardly long time before completing what he wanted me to know about the visit to the doctor's office. "The doctor said he really thinks it's Alzheimer's, but there will be more tests and such." His voice didn't change, but Mr. Dell seemed to have difficulty getting his words out. "He wants me to encourage her to remain as active as possible. He said he will start her on some medication that may help with the symptoms, but it won't necessarily stop her from developing the bad part of Alzheimer's. You know, the full-blown part." He lowered his head slightly and looked toward the floor before speaking again. "The doctor said he doesn't know how fast or how slow it will progress."

He looked up at me with questioning eyes. "I took the way he said that—how fast or how slow—as really meaning that it will progress. That's what he was trying to get us to understand, isn't it? That it's going to get worse."

He looked sad, and the only way I could respond was with a soft nod of my head in agreement with his conclusion. I knew he realized he was going to be losing a large part of the joy in his life.

By the second appointment, the other possibilities for her symptoms had been ruled out, and the doctor explained to both Mr. and Mrs. Dell that additional testing and follow-up evaluations could be done if they liked. Mr. Dell asked if doing so would change the course. "Not really. You discuss it and let me know. In the meantime, we'll just call it probable Alzheimer's disease—early stage."

Mr. Dell explained that the doctor did not offer hope for her to get better. "He basically said, 'It has happened, and you can't stop it. Perhaps we can slow it down—somewhat.' A runaway freight train is what I thought of."

As Mr. Dell talked, thoughts bombarded my mind, thoughts like a day would come when she would lose her ability to remember how to get to the grocery store, when she would forget what day it was or what she was supposed to do. And one thing would be certain: she wouldn't get her memory back with any medication the doctor gave her. Nothing would bring those dead neurons back to life. The damage was done.

I hated to hear what Mrs. Dell's doctor had to say about Alzheimer's, but I was thankful it awoke me to a medical realization. It made me realize that prevention is the answer.

Those initial twenty years when it is developing are the prime time to go to battle. But even if you find yourself in the next stage, when you realize you are not remembering a name, or forgetting where you placed something, or not being able to reason or process something you used to do—that is also the time to commit to prevention. That is also the time to learn what you can do to decrease your chances of ever being told, "Take this medicine—it won't cure it or prevent it from progressing but it may help with your symptoms."

Fight to prevent any beta-amyloid plaque formation. Fight even if there is some plaque but no symptoms—yet. And yes, fight it even if symptoms have arrived. Fight its progression all the way to the ground.

Stage 3

Stage 3 is called dementia due to Alzheimer's disease. Stage 3 involves noticeable memory problems, and a person's thinking and reasoning affect their behavior to the point that they have to depend on someone else to help with everyday activities. When we speak of dementia, we are talking about stage 3 Alzheimer's.

On the dreadful day a person goes from stage 2 MCI to stage 3 Alzheimer's dementia, they are no longer able to perform the activities of a normal day without assistance from someone else. The day they are told they can no longer drive is a common initial realization of Stage 3. They soon will not be able to make breakfast, decide what to wear, or even dress themselves. All their familiar habits, previously enjoyed, will become foreign to them.

The Scary Numbers

Have you visited a nursing home recently? If not, I suggest you visit one and walk down the hallway. As you do, think about some of the statistics from the Alzheimer's Association's publication "Alzheimer's Disease Facts and Figures." *Seventy-five percent of nursing home admissions for people over age eighty are due to Alzheimer's.* Two-thirds of those who die of dementia do so in nursing homes. Once the diagnosis of Alzheimer's is made, 40 percent of a person's remaining life will be spent in a nursing home setting. The contributing causes of death for people with Alzheimer's are most often pneumonia and urinary tract infections. They get pneumonia because they have a slight stroke that affects their swallowing, and some of their saliva incorrectly goes down their trachea into their lungs rather than down their esophagus. According to Medicare data, one-third of all seniors who die in a given year have been diagnosed with Alzheimer's dementia. About half of all people who visit a doctor for memory symptoms will develop stage 3 dementia in three to four years.

Most people know that heart attacks and strokes kill more Americans than any other cause. But few realize that dementia is the second largest contributor to death behind heart failure.

The last of the scary numbers is that most people who develop Alzheimer's live four to eight years in stage 2 and stage 3 of the disease.

When Mrs. Dell returned home that day after being presented with the reality of her diagnosis, Mr. Dell said she sat and stared out the sliding glass door for a long time. I couldn't help but wonder, was she thinking about her future, when she wouldn't be able to remember anything, like when her mother developed Alzheimer's?

I couldn't bring myself to tell Mr. Dell that the medical literature pointed out that nearly half of all people who visit a doctor concerning symptoms such as those Mrs. Dell presented with develop full-blown Alzheimer's dementia within three to four years. Some things are better left unsaid.

3

The Brain, Imagery, and Testing

Alzheimer's Markers

To understand what happens in the brain of someone with Alzheimer's, let's look at the neuron—the nerve cell itself. In a brain affected by Alzheimer's, a war is ongoing. In different sections of the brain, clumps of neurons are slowly being destroyed. It's the bad army versus the good. The bad is associated with Alzheimer's disease. The good cells keep thoughts and actions and memory going until the bad begin winning more and more of the battles. The ultimate diagnosis is made at an autopsy when the brain is dissected and sliced into thin strips that can be examined under a microscope.

The brain normally produces beta-amyloid protein. It also routinely removes old beta-amyloid as new protein is produced. An extremely accurate mechanism around the nerve cells of the brain controls the production and the elimination of beta-amyloid. But in Alzheimer's patients, the excess beta-amyloid is not completely removed. It doesn't flow through the controlling barrier into the bloodstream as it should. A healthy brain has about one hundred billion brain cells. Each of these neurons has long, branching extensions that enable the neuron to form specialized connections with surrounding nerve cells. These connections are called synapses. There are an estimated one hundred trillion starfish-like fingers extending out from neurons that end as synapses. Information flows in tiny bursts of chemicals that are released by one nerve cell and detected by a receiving neuron.

As long as the normal amount of beta-amyloid is floating around in the fluid surrounding each cell, or neuron, information can be transferred rapidly and consistently. Everything works properly. Memory, thoughts, emotions, skills, and body movements are under control. When Alzheimer's begins to develop, however, the excess beta-amyloid begins to accumulate and gel. The surrounding fluid becomes filled more and more with the sticky substance until it thickens enough to become a plaque. This plaque interferes with the synapses that pass information from one cell to another. When this happens, the neurons begin to die and shrink in size. The result is a loss of volume of brain tissue.

A second protein fits into the picture of Alzheimer's: tau protein. It is located inside the neuron itself and is important in sending messages from one brain cell to another. Inside each neuron are pathways like railroad tracks with multiple branching extensions. The neuron is constantly moving food and other nutrients along these tracks. The tau protein located inside the neuron's system keeps these tracks lined up in straight rows so they can function properly. As beta-amyloid plaques collect on the outside of the brain cells, tau protein begins to malfunction and sticks together, forming tangles within the cell. These tangles cause the tracks to fall apart and block the transport of essential nutrients throughout the inside of the neuron. They also block the transfer of messages from one neuron to another at the synapses, adding to the cause of death of the brain cell.

As the production of beta-amyloid plaques and tau tangles progresses and more and more brain cells die, the brain begins to shrink in volume. In brain studies of people with advanced Alzheimer's, different areas of the brain show significant shrinkage due to cells dying off. Also visible are piles of rubbish consisting of beta-amyloid plaques and dying and dead neurons. This graveyard is the telltale sign of Alzheimer's. But it is complex. There are many factors that play into the complicated process called Alzheimer's. Alzheimer's is not simply the accumulation of the beta-amyloid. There are a multitude of other factors in the equation.

I kept a small cartoon on my desk for years. It was a picture of two vagrants sitting on a park bench. Both were leaning back, one with his hands behind his head. He had his legs straight out in front of him with his feet crossed. There was a large hole in each sole of his shoes. The caption read: "My father said you had to spend money to make money—but obviously, there's more to it than that."

Obviously, there's more to Alzheimer's than just the accumulation of beta-amyloid plaques and tau tangles. For example, we do not yet know what causes the process to begin. In addition, autopsies have revealed that individuals who were completely intact from a mental standpoint, with no symptoms of Alzheimer's, had beta-amyloid plaques and tau tangles in their brains. Studies show that *up to one-third of older people who are considered normal have some deposits of beta-amyloid within the brain.* Further, around 80 percent of people diagnosed with Alzheimer's also have disease in the arteries going to or within the brain.

Clearly, Alzheimer's is a complex disease, and people must do everything they can to decrease their risk. Later in this book, you'll learn what you can do to protect your brain against Alzheimer's.

The Effect of Alzheimer's on the Brain

The longer the Alzheimer's process goes on, the more beta-amyloid plaques that form and the more nerve cells that die, resulting in less volume of active brain mass.

We will break down the brain tissue into three components in order to show what happens as Alzheimer's sets in. The most significant part of the brain that affects memory is the hippocampus. This area is relatively small and is situated near the base of the brain structure. It is most important in short-term memory. In early Alzheimer's, an individual may lose this short-term memory but be able to remember distinctly things that happened many years ago.

The second area of the brain is called the cortex. This part of the brain also plays an important role in memory but is more utilized in long-term memory as well as the thinking process. The cortex is the quarter-inch outer covering of the brain. It contains billions of neurons and accounts for approximately 40 percent of the brain's tissue.

The third area affected by Alzheimer's is the ventricles. These cavities are filled with clear liquid called cerebrospinal fluid, which travels down the spinal canal and performs many functions in the central nervous system.

A normal, healthy brain has a normal-sized hippocampus, normal thickness of the cortex, and a normal volume of fluid in the ventricles. As Alzheimer's progresses, more and more beta-amyloid plaques form, along with tau tangles, and the neurons begin to die. As they do so, that area of the brain shrinks and the ventricles make up for the loss in brain mass by filling up with fluid, which causes them to increase in size.

The first part of the brain involved in Alzheimer's is usually the hippocampus, with the associated short-term memory loss. The second area is often the cortex, which involves the memory and also a person's ability to keep a normal attention span and to reason properly. Language control is also affected.

As the disease continues to progress, more deposits of beta-amyloid form, the brain tissue continues to shrink, and the ventricles enlarge even more. The brain becomes less and less dense as the Alzheimer's process worsens.

The Secret Disease

Researchers state that Alzheimer's begins many years before the first symptom appears, sometimes twenty or even thirty years before a person exhibits symptoms.

What scientific evidence do they have that something is going on that far ahead of symptoms?

First, brain-imaging studies confirm the existence of beta-amyloid plaques in people without Alzheimer's symptoms. In fact, *up to a third of people over age sixty-five already have these plaques beginning to develop in their brains.*

Research has also shown that as cells die in the brain because of beta-amyloid plaques, that particular part of the brain gets smaller because fewer full-sized, healthy cells remain. Both beta-amyloid plaques and the shrinkage of brain volume are visible on MRIs and PET scans before the onset of symptoms.

MRI stands for magnetic resonance imaging. An MRI provides a detailed picture of the brain without the use of X-ray radiation. It works because hydrogen atoms in the brain are affected by rotating a powerful magnet around a person's head. There is even a more specialized type of MRI that can detect if a certain part of the brain is presently active. This can test activity going on in the brain while someone is taking one of the mental tests to evaluate the progress of their

Alzheimer's. The MRI can tell if a certain part of the brain is functioning while the individual is memorizing a list of words or numbers to recall or similar questions on the test. The MRI is a very beneficial type of imaging study of your brain. Think of a loaf of bread with multiple slices stacked side by side. An MRI provides pictures of multiple slices of brain tissue. Such pictures reveal how much of a slice is brain tissue and how much is fluid. They can measure whether a portion of brain mass is of normal size or if it is shrinking, as seen in Alzheimer's. If an area shows shrinkage, it can be followed by subsequent MRIs to see any progression of deterioration of that area.

PET stands for positron emission tomography. This scan traces blood flow and energy usage in the brain. In a PET scan, special molecules are tagged with a radioactive substance and injected into a person's vein. The injected material goes to the beta-amyloid and attaches itself to it. Doctors can actually see where the accumulation of this sticky plaque is forming.

Researchers combined their findings from brain-imaging studies with mental testing and found that as more beta-amyloid built up, mental test scores worsened. This too was seen before any symptoms, before an individual knew anything was going on in their brain. Even though the mental test scores were worsening, the disease process was not bad enough to cause any noticeable symptoms. Many cells were being killed in the battle, but enough healthy cells remained to allow the person to continue functioning normally. *The brain-imaging studies combined with the mental test scores leave little doubt in my mind: the process of Alzheimer's can begin without a person even knowing it.*

Mrs. Dell didn't have all the brain studies to prove her diagnosis of Alzheimer's. I would like to believe she would have been encouraged to change some of her lifestyle habits if she had been shown pictures of an MRI study or a PET scan of her brain. Perhaps she would have begun an exercise program or changed her eating habits or lost weight. But her diagnosis of probable Alzheimer's didn't seem to affect her all that much. She continued being as active as she had been before the diagnosis. She still sang at church, although now she sat in the auditorium rather than in the choir loft. The flowers in her yard remained the central point in her life. She hosted the supper club group at her home whenever it was her turn. The only thing that changed was, now Mr. Dell did the cooking. He said she either lost interest in cooking or didn't seem to be able to do it anymore. "Even with a recipe," he would say.

Tracing the Progression of Alzheimer's

Researchers can follow an individual and watch the buildup of beta-amyloid plaques and the decreasing volume of certain parts of the brain as the symptoms of Alzheimer's develop and progress.

An article published in the *Journal of the American Medical Association Neurology* revealed that as brain studies show more signs of Alzheimer's, symptoms worsen. The study looked at fifty-four healthy elderly individuals who had some beta-amyloid in their brains but no symptoms. They all underwent MRI imaging and PET scans to evaluate their brains. They also underwent verbal and written tests to determine their memory ability as well as other mental functions. So this was a fairly extensive study to evaluate the correlation between the verbal and written testing for Alzheimer's with imaging studies on the brain. The question the study wanted to answer is whether the people with the Alzheimer's findings on the brain-imaging studies did worse on their mental testing, and if the follow-up scans worsened, did the mental test results worsen also? These people were evaluated one and a half years and three years later. As the MRIs and PET scans showed a worsening of the beta-amyloid plaques and more shrinkage of brain tissue, the mental test results also worsened.

The Australian Imaging Biomarkers and Lifestyle Rate of Change Study was performed on forty-four healthy older adults. Studies were done to see what amount of beta-amyloid formation was found in the brains of these subjects. They were also given memory and thinking tests at the beginning of the study and then again six months later when imaging studies of their brains were repeated. The group was divided into two subgroups. One group had low levels of beta-amyloid in their brains at the beginning of the study, and the other group was composed of individuals who had higher levels of beta-amyloid.

The study showed that the *participants with higher levels of beta-amyloid experienced a greater decline in their memory and thinking tests than those with the low levels of beta-amyloid.*

The same Australian group reported a study in the medical journal *Neurology* that showed similar findings. These individuals were healthy adults with a mean age of seventy-six who were normal from a neurological standpoint. In other words, they showed no signs or symptoms of Alzheimer's. Yet their PET scans showed beta-amyloid buildup in parts of their brains.

Memory and verbal tests were repeated eighteen months later, as were PET scans. Those with high beta-amyloid levels, as compared to those with low amounts, showed "significantly greater decline in working memory and verbal and visual episodic memory at 18 months." In other words, those with more beta-amyloid plaques in their brains scored worse on their memory and thinking tests than those with fewer beta-amyloid plaques. The study showed the correlation between the greater amount of beta-amyloid and the worsening on their mental test scores. Remember, these were all asymptomatic people who would not have known they were in stage 1 of Alzheimer's had they not had the imaging scans done of their brains. They showed no signs of Alzheimer's or any other dementia. These were what we would call "normal" adults, going along with their daily routine similar to what

Mrs. Dell was doing for the twenty years prior to her initial symptom of forgetfulness.

The beginning of Alzheimer's could be happening right now in your brain without a clue or warning. Several studies utilizing PET scans have shown that approximately one-third of healthy elderly people have significant beta-amyloid deposition within their brains without having symptoms. That means a third of the participants had stage 1 Alzheimer's and didn't know it—yet.

When would she tell her friends? When would she explain to her grandchildren? What would she say to them? She wanted her relationships with them to stay the same. Life was not all that different than before her diagnosis. Why discuss it with anyone? Why not just live life one day at a time? Mrs. Dell knew one bit of her life would persist no matter what: her friends at supper club. The supper club couples had met in each member's home for years. They made her smile. No matter how much the disease whittled her away, she knew they would be loyal to the end.

Tests for Alzheimer's

The doctor gave Mrs. Dell the diagnosis of probable Alzheimer's—early stage. Back then the word *probable* was used because a definitive diagnosis could not be made until an autopsy was performed and a pathologist looked at a piece of brain tissue under a microscope. Now the word *probable* may still be used, but the exciting news is that tests can be performed to reveal the overall probability of the disease. In addition to MRIs and PET scans, which we already discussed, doctors can perform a test involving the cerebrospinal fluid. A doctor places a needle into the spinal area and draws off some cerebrospinal fluid. This fluid can indicate how much beta-amyloid is in the fluid of the brain area. If a lot of beta-amyloid is being retained in the brain area and it is forming plaque, then there is less in the spinal area.

Mental testing is also often performed. If a patient like Mrs. Dell goes to their doctor complaining of memory problems, they most likely take one of several standard tests. As time progresses, the patients who have Alzheimer's remember less and less, are unable to respond to specific instructions, and are unable to perform as well on the test as they did previously.

Let's say you took your mother in for an examination. The doctor might say, "I am going to tell you someone's name and their address. After I tell you, I want you to repeat it back to me so I know you understood what I said. I want you to remember this name and address because I am going to ask you to repeat it back to me in a few minutes." The doctor says something like, "Jim Greene, 39 East Street, Kingston." The doctor asks her to repeat it several times to make sure she has it right.

Then the doctor asks a question related to orientation to time such as, "What is today's date? What is the day, the month, and the year?" If she answers correctly, she receives a point.

The next question centers on her visual concept of space. She is handed a blank piece of paper and instructed to draw a clock with all the numbers in the correct place and evenly spaced. If she spaces the numbers properly, she is given another point.

Third, she is instructed to draw the hands on the clock to represent five minutes before two o'clock. She is credited a point if she does this properly.

Next the doctor asks her to relate something specific that occurred in the news in the past week. She receives another point if she can do so.

Then the big memory question comes to the forefront. She is asked to repeat the name and address she was given at the beginning of the exam. She is given a point if she recalls "Jim," another point for "Greene," another for "39," another for "East Street," and another for "Kingston."

The test has a total of nine points. If she gets all nine, she is considered normal from a mental and reasoning standpoint, and no further testing is required. However, if her score is between five and eight, the doctor will want more information and will ask you several questions about whether you think your mother has changed mentally.

Does she have more difficulty remembering things that happened recently than she used to? Is she having more trouble recalling conversations a few days later? Is she having trouble finding the right word to complete a sentence?

Is she less able to pay bills or keep up with her finances? If she is on medication, is she less able to take it properly by herself? Does she need assistance with driving and making decisions?

If you answer yes to one to three questions, then her cognition is in question and additional studies will take place to rule out other causes of the problem. Then tests for Alzheimer's become the focus.

There are different tests and questions, and this example gives you an idea of what may be asked.

In summary, spinal tap and some blood studies may be helpful, but Alzheimer's shows its progress best through MRI, PET, and/or mental testing first by the accumulation of beta-amyloid, followed by the accumulation of the tau tangles, then the dying of neurons with resultant shrinkage of brain mass. And then you have symptoms.

But in those days, it was not routine for such tests to be done. No MRIs or PET scans or drawing of spinal fluid. Just the clinical diagnosis of what was developing, which was becoming obvious to her doctor—as well as Mrs. Dell's family and some close friends.

Even though she didn't seem to realize she was getting confused, she was. She kept losing her earrings. Her favorite key chain kept disappearing, but she would eventually find it. "I've always had trouble keeping up with my keys," was her usual response. Little threads that held her mind together were breaking, but nothing had begun to unravel. She had convinced herself she was going to stay who she was—for as long as possible.

The Most Exciting News Concerning Alzheimer's

These new tests are so exciting because we are now able to measure the beta-amyloid in the brain and see if developing certain lifestyles makes a difference. Will people who exercise have less beta-amyloid than those who don't? What about people who eat healthy or are at their ideal weight compared to people who are overweight or don't eat properly? It is even more exciting to realize our beliefs about Alzheimer's dementia have shifted from the belief that it is an untreatable and almost inevitable aspect of aging to a potentially preventable problem.

To me, *these studies of the brain are the most significant advances in being able to study whether avoiding certain risk factors can change your chances of developing Alzheimer's.* Scientists can take a group of people who exercise a certain measured amount of exertion and compare them to a group of couch potatoes who are completely sedentary and follow them for several years. What they are seeing on the imaging studies is that beta-amyloid is building up in the brains of the ones who don't exercise, while the ones who do don't have the buildup of the plaques. It's a great wake-up call to those who are willing to commit to changing their lifestyles.

There are similar findings with certain diets as compared to others. Previous studies include people who are overweight or have high blood pressure or diabetes. The results show that people with these risk factors have a progressive increase in the beta-amyloid buildup in comparison to individuals who do not have such risk factors.

So the bottom line is this: go to war on the factors that are commonly found in the groups of Alzheimer's patients and develop the habits of the group that doesn't have the dreaded disease.

It is encouraging to know Alzheimer's can be detected early and followed through to the last step of the disease, but it is also good to know what can be done to prevent it from happening or to slow its progress down to a crawl.

In summary, think of MRI imaging as being able to let us see an area of the brain that has been affected by Alzheimer's where a significant number of cells have died, leaving less volume of brain tissue in that area. The MRI clearly shows the shrinkage.

Think of PET scans as being able to actually see where beta-amyloid plaques are present.

Should You Be Tested?

I asked a friend who was completely asymptomatic for Alzheimer's if he would change his lifestyle habits if MRI imaging or a PET scan showed that he had beta-amyloid plaques beginning to form in his brain. He said if he knew he was developing the buildup of what causes the disease, he would definitely do something about it.

I wanted to make a point with him. Scans can detect the disease process before there are any symptoms. But even if my friend tested positive for Alzheimer's, no medical treatment could cure the damage already done. His only way to fight is by changing how he lives now.

The question I want you to seriously consider is this: Would you change your lifestyle habits if you found out beta-amyloid plaques were forming in your brain? Just a few plaques? Or a lot of plaques? What if doctors discovered with an MRI that the hippocampus of your brain had decreased in size? That would mean enough beta-amyloid plaques were present to cause the death of enough cells so that the volume of brain tissue in that small area had begun to decline. Would abnormal findings spur you into doing something about decreasing your chances of getting Alzheimer's?

Here's my point. Why in the world would anyone wait for a brain study that showed the beginning of Alzheimer's before deciding to do something to help prevent it? *That is like waiting until you cough up blood from a lung tumor before deciding to quit smoking.* Don't wait until you begin forgetting things to address the risk factors so prevalent in Alzheimer's patients.

My guess is that you don't need a scan of your brain to make you take action to improve your health. It is something we all ought to decide—that we want the healthiest body we can possibly have, no matter what a brain scan may show. Health ought to be our number-one priority. This is the only body we receive. It is going to either run at peak performance or function at a less-than-optimum setting, just like your car. You decide whether you are going to change the oil and keep the tires inflated. You decide what type of gasoline you are going to use. This book gives you knowledge and motivation so you will have both the desire and the commitment to keep your most prized possession running at the highest level possible.

Since there is no cure for Alzheimer's, more studies are exploring ways to prevent the disease. Prevention is the only "cure." Later in this book, we will address the things you can do to prevent the risks that are known to cause and worsen Alzheimer's.

Common sense tells us to take charge of what we can control. So many studies on prevention show the correlation between the health of the arteries of the heart and the health of the arteries of the brain. The medical studies tell us that what is good for the heart is good for the brain. Research has proven that specific lifestyle changes improve the health of the heart. Now studies show that the vascular risk factors that increase the risk of a heart attack are the same vascular risk factors that increase the risk of Alzheimer's. An article in the journal *Clinical Science* puts it best: *aggressive treatment of these vascular risk factors for the prevention of Alzheimer's disease appears warranted and should be vigorously pursued.*

Even if symptoms have begun, you want the disease to progress as slowly as possible. As stated in an article in *Acta Neuropathologica*, these vascular risk factors "accelerate the tempo of the dementia." You don't want symptoms to accelerate; you want to do everything you can to stop them in their tracks. So before we look at the lifestyle risk factors for Alzheimer's and how to avoid them, we need to address the role arteries play in Alzheimer's.

I knew the diagnosis her doctor had given. I understood what was on the horizon, soon to become reality. But did she? Did she comprehend what was beginning and the eventual dreaded end? Could she see herself ending up like her mother? If she did, she didn't seem to be admitting it to herself. She acted as if everything was normal. She still watered her flowers, paid the bills, and went to the grocery store almost every day. She watched the news and *Jeopardy* on television every night. She still smiled, was still so pleasant. What did she know, and what did she think?

The last time I had visited them, Mr. Dell told me he noticed that Mrs. Dell seemed to be having more trouble keeping track of her car keys. "So I placed a special little bowl on the side table just as you enter the house from the patio. I told her to put the car keys in the bowl every time she came home and they would always be in the bowl when she got ready to leave the next time. She actually thanked me, got her keys out of her purse, and placed them in the bowl." Mr. Dell smiled.

"But she told me the other day she couldn't find her keys. She asked me if I had hidden them. Can you believe that? I reminded her that if she put them in the bowl, they would always be there when she needed them. She just looked at me and said, 'I know, but I forgot.'"

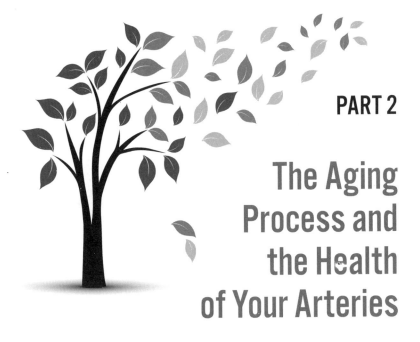

PART 2

The Aging Process and the Health of Your Arteries

4

The Importance
of Protecting Your Arteries

Memorize this statement: *a healthy brain depends on the health of the heart as well as the arteries of the heart and the brain.*

Nerve cells have no energy reserves, and their performance of mental tasks is critically dependent on the steady delivery of oxygen and nutrients through the blood. When this delivery system is inadequate, the brain suffers.

To understand the heart-brain connection, let's look at the system of blood flow that supplies the individual neurons in the brain.

Every time your heart beats, 20 to 25 percent of the blood propelled out of your heart goes to your brain. Your brain needs one quarter of your blood supply. Your heart and arteries play a crucial role in keeping your brain functioning at peak performance. Consider the impact of your brain not getting enough blood flow. An *Archives of Neurology* article reports that within three years after a stroke, 23 percent of the individuals will develop dementia.

In reviewing the medical literature, I find it remarkable how many articles use the phrase "What is good for the heart is good for the brain." The lifestyle practices that lead to heart disease are the same ones found in patients with Alzheimer's. The risk factors that affect both heart disease and Alzheimer's include high lethal LDL cholesterol that affects your arteries in your heart as well as your brain, being overweight or obese, being inactive, having high blood pressure, and having diabetes.

"I am not going to go on a diet," Mrs. Dell said. "I have always eaten what I want, and I am going to continue. And I am not going to exercise. I will take care of my flowers like I have for years and will keep enjoying doing it. You are not going to get me to run every day, and I don't care what you say." That was the end of the discussion.

However, she did agree to take the medicine her doctor prescribed.

It was about three months before my next visit. Mr. Dell didn't think she should be driving. He was afraid she would get lost or maybe even hurt somebody. "She won't listen to me. Can you tell her?" I told him I would do what I could.

My conversation with Mrs. Dell was like talking to a doorpost. "I can drive just fine," she said, and that was that.

The System of Blood Flow to the Brain

The heart and the larger arteries pump blood to the brain. The two main arteries are the carotid arteries in the neck. As I mentioned earlier, every time the heart beats, 20 to 25 percent of the blood propelled out of the heart goes to the brain. The brain is only 2 percent of the body's total weight, but the brain utilizes 20 percent of the oxygen we breathe and 20 percent of the nutrients we take in from food. This shows how important the heart and larger arteries are for getting the needed oxygen and nutrients to each neuron of the brain.

But smaller arteries also have an important role. The small arteries within the brain have two major functions. The first is delivering oxygen and nutrients *to* the brain cells. The other function is equally important. It is the removal of waste products *from* the brain.

The questions kept coming to mind. How long does stage 2 last before progressing to stage 3, where she loses her independence? What tips the scale to stage 3? When does her stage 3 begin? When will she have to depend on someone else to help get through the day? When will Mr. Dell have to take her car keys away from her? I had been thinking about the Dells and wondering how long they would be able to remain in their present home. There would be two possibilities: either caregivers at home or a move to some type of extended-care facility. Even though Mrs. Dell was living a fairly normal life,

I wondered if she thought about the future. Did they talk about long-term care?

She and Mr. Dell agreed to go and have a look. They visited an extremely nice retirement center that had an assisted-living section and an extended-care facility. They would live in a fairly small but attractive separate home, which they would buy. And when Mrs. Dell needed more attention, she would be transferred to a private room where all her needs would be taken care of.

She would be seen every day, meals prepared, bed linen washed. Everything taken care of. The last building they toured had single rooms where total care could be given. Fed, bathed, teeth brushed. The money they would pay for the home would be donated to the care facility once they both passed, but each would be taken care of for the rest of their lives. It seemed an ideal setup for both of them. However, on the way home when Mrs. Dell was asked what her thoughts were, she gave a short reply. "It is a very nice facility, but I would like to live in our house for as long as possible." She hesitated a moment before mentioning, "That last room—I wouldn't ever want to be there."

I realized it was time to begin looking for a caregiver to start spending time with her, perhaps just during the day at first. Mr. Dell could take care of the nights and weekends. But she needed someone who could be there for her Monday through Friday.

Arterial Disease and the Brain

Disease of the arteries in three areas of the body can have an effect on the brain:

1. The arteries of the heart
2. The arteries that feed the brain, especially the carotid arteries in the neck
3. The small arteries within the brain

The term used when talking about disease or plaque in the main arteries leading to the brain is *atherosclerosis*. Disease of the arteries in the brain is called *cerebrovascular disease*.

When my grandfather was a young man, he was walking home along the railroad tracks and noticed a switch was thrown in such a way that an oncoming train would derail. Knowing there was a train coming in the next ten minutes, he immediately began running up the tracks to warn the engineer. He was able to flag down the train in time for it to stop before it reached the switch. He prevented a derailment and possibly saved many lives. For that deed, the Southern Railroad offered him a job for life.

I was in the fifth grade when my family moved to a different state. After a year, we returned for a visit. I was so excited to surprise my grandfather. I could barely run fast enough around the side of their home. I saw him sitting on the low rock wall, a small tree stump directly in front of him. He was holding a small ax in his right hand and a piece of wood in his left. He was cutting the wood into kindling, one stroke of the ax after another. My grandfather, my lifelong hero, asked me, "Are you the boy who stole my wheelbarrow?" He took one more chop and then just stared at me, waiting for an answer.

My grandmother was a few steps behind me and spoke only a simple sentence. "Oh, Ben, that's one of Amy's boys." Then she put her arm around my waist and led me into the house. Once inside, her explanation was one she thought I would understand. But I had no idea what she was talking about, nor would I understand until I entered medical school and studied anatomy. Her comment was, "Don't pay any attention to him. He has hardening of the arteries."

What my grandmother was saying about my grandfather was that he had Alzheimer's dementia. Back then they didn't call it Alzheimer's dementia or vascular dementia. They called it hardening of the arteries. If these people went to their doctor, problems related to their arteries became evident. Perhaps the doctor could feel a vibrating sensation when examining the carotid artery. Checking the two arteries that run up the front sides of the neck on each side of the trachea has been routine since physicians first began doing physical examinations. It is part of the routine physical examination taught to first-year students in medical school. Students also take their newly acquired stethoscope and listen to these two arteries. The professor will explain why such an exam is essential. The two carotid arteries are the main conduit supplying the brain with the needed blood flow carrying essential oxygen and nutrients. If there is a partial blockage, the turbulent movement of the blood hitting the blockage can be palpated by the medical student's fingertips. With a smaller blockage, the stethoscope will pick up an audible swishing sound with each beat of the heart. A partial blockage can be operated on and removed or even possibly stented.

I was too young to understand whether my grandfather had a hardened carotid artery or not, but as the years passed, I recognized that the disease of his arteries most likely played a role in his dementia. An article in *Aging Research Reviews* pointed out that numerous clinical studies concluded that *heart disease and blockage of carotid arteries are major risk factors for cognitive mental decline.*

The bottom line is that the brain requires an abundance of oxygen and nutrients to function properly. Progressive damage to the arteries over the years impedes the flow of oxygen-rich blood that each cell needs to function. New research connects a decrease in the amount of blood that the heart pumps with each beat to an increase in the risk of memory loss and a progression to Alzheimer's dementia. These studies correlate an unhealthy heart with an unhealthy brain, resulting in dementia.

This was emphasized in a key statement in an article published in the journal *Circulation*. "More people need to know about the connection between vascular disease and dementia." The one statement that I liked best concerned the connection between disease of our arteries and dementia: "The key to all this is prevention." The best action you can take to protect your brain is to develop the three lifestyles that show reduced odds of developing the disease. Other medical journal articles highlight the correlation between the health of the arteries and the health of the brain. One interesting study pointed out that because the brain utilizes such a high proportion of total blood flow throughout the body, it is pretty obvious that *anything that affects the arteries carrying that high amount of blood to the brain will also affect how the brain functions.*

The Diabetes Heart Study studied the correlation between the health of the heart and the scores on mental testing used to evaluate a person's cognition in relation to symptoms that could lead to Alzheimer's. Here is what researchers found.

Before symptoms were apparent, researchers measured the amount of plaque within the arterial walls of the arteries in the heart. Then seven years later, they gave the same individuals mental tests that measured memory, executive function, and how fast they processed different situations. The study found that the individuals with more plaque when the study began scored lower on the mental tests than the people with the least amount of plaque in the arteries in their hearts.

It is fairly easy to understand that if the arteries of the heart are diseased, the heart is going to pump less efficiently. It also makes sense that if there are diseased arteries due to plaque formation and inflammation, there will be less blood flow to the brain. An interesting article published in the journal *Neurology* makes it a little easier to understand the importance of blood flow in the brain network. The arterial system may play a significant role in the beta-amyloid accumulation in the brain. The arteries in the brain have two major functions. The first we have mentioned: delivering oxygen and nutrients to the brain cells. But the other purpose is equally important. That is the removal of the waste products of the brain. There are little channels along the pathways of the arteries that eliminate extra fluid from around the cells as well as removing waste-type products that include excess beta-amyloid. Alzheimer's disease is characterized by the failure of the elimination of the tau that ends up in the tau tangles, as well as the removal of beta-amyloid.

I don't want to get too deep into the structure of how the brain is supplied by your arteries, but this is a little anatomy lesson that will help you understand what could be happening to cause the beta-amyloid accumulation that is seen in Alzheimer's. It also gives you insight as to why it is so important to do what is necessary to keep your arteries healthy by living the proper lifestyles.

The arterial system gets smaller and smaller, ending up at the neurons, the working cells of the brain. This is where there are barriers between the minute arterial structure and the neurons. These dividing walls, or barriers, are called the *blood-brain barriers*. They are extremely important in the transferring of oxygen and nutrients from the bloodstream into the neurons and their surrounding fluid. The barriers are equally important in allowing waste products from within the surrounding fluid to enter back into the bloodstream to be carried away. Such products include excess beta-amyloid. The blood-brain barriers need to be working properly to get oxygen and nutrients in and waste products out. If the beta-amyloid can't get out through the barriers, the result is excess beta-amyloid remaining around the brain cells. As you know, excess beta-amyloid leads to beta-amyloid plaques, which are the hallmark of Alzheimer's.

I explain this little bit of minute detail so you can understand that if this blood-brain barrier is not functioning properly, there is a detrimental association resulting in an increase of the symptoms of Alzheimer's. The health of your arteries is vital in the proper functioning of this blood-brain barrier.

The report in *Neurology* also noted that disease and plaque formation in the larger carotid arteries results in low blood flow damage that can result in either a full-blown stroke or the mini-strokes that happen but don't cause symptoms. If you want to feel one of these arteries, take your finger and feel just to one side or the other of your neck just beside your windpipe. That's your carotid artery. That's one of the arteries researchers talk about when comparing the larger arteries with the smaller ones.

A good friend of mine called me the other day and told me the doctors had just done a test that showed one of his carotids was 60 percent blocked. He had no idea anything was wrong. He changed his eating habits that day and decided to exercise more than simply playing golf four times a week as he was previously doing.

A study reported in *Neurology* did not focus on the large carotid arteries that supply the brain but rather the micro-arteries within the brain. You can't feel these small arteries. As a matter of fact, you need a microscope to see them. These tiny arteries are where the blood-brain barriers are located. Arterial disease in these tiny areas was shown to cause a malfunction of the blood-brain barriers, affecting the removal of fluids and waste from the brains of people with Alzheimer's. So even the walls of these tiny arteries can be affected similar to the way the larger carotid arteries are affected by plaque. Instead of plaque buildup in the walls of these small arteries, there is an increase in fibrous tissue that hampers their function. The study concluded that the exact cause of the beta-amyloid problem is not known, but the health of the arterial system may play a significant role in Alzheimer's by affecting the drainage aspect of the blood-brain barriers.

The health of the arteries is extremely important, so bear with me as we quickly go over one more study concerning how disease of the arteries may play a role in the cause of Alzheimer's. It was published in the medical journal *Hypertension* and was based on microscopic autopsy findings concerning the health of the arterial system around the nerve cells and the accumulation of beta-amyloid around those cells. The findings showed that beta-amyloid, in conjunction with high blood pressure, greatly weakened the micro-arterial walls around the blood-brain barriers, which resulted in reduced beta-amyloid clearance from the brain. This raises the question: Is the main cause of Alzheimer's the beta-amyloid or the health of the arterial system that controls how much blood is supplied to the brain-cell complexes? Any way you look at it, *the health of the arteries plays a significant role in Alzheimer's.*

Here is another important point from this study. You know that excess weight or obesity affects the health of the arteries. The report showed that being overweight or obese in midlife correlated with a lower functioning of the blood-brain barriers almost twenty-five years later. Being inactive affects the health of those arteries, and eating the wrong foods results in damage to those arteries. All three of these are called risk factors. You are going to learn exactly how to fight all three of these arterial risk factors to win the battle even before it starts.

Special MRI studies can detect how much blood flow is happening in the brain. One such study, published in the *Annals of Neurology*, used MRIs to measure the flow of blood as well as the size of parts of the brain. Researchers gave almost eight thousand people base testing for cognition, which involved thinking, reasoning, and memory. The age of the participants was fifty-five and above. *The participants with greater blood flow in the brain were less likely to have Alzheimer's dementia.* The individuals with better blood flow scored higher on the mental testing, and the size of their hippocampuses was significantly larger as seen on MRIs. The area of the brain that is the most susceptible to a decrease in blood flow due to disease of the arteries is the hippocampus. And the hippocampus is also one of the earliest areas of the brain affected by Alzheimer's disease. The study concluded that *the factors that cause a risk to the health of your arteries play a significant role in the cause of developing Alzheimer's dementia as well as a faster decline once someone first develops dementia.*

The takeaway of the study is that decrease in blood flow to the brain is very significant and the arterial risk factors that result in the decreased blood flow are preventable. I will emphasize again: *your aging process is determined by the health of your arteries.* You have control of how you take care of your body. No one else determines whether you exercise or not. No one controls what you choose to eat. You are the only one who can determine if you are going to lose weight and develop a lifestyle that lets you maintain that weight.

I reiterate another study that revealed the impact of the brain not getting enough blood. An *Archives of Neurology* article reported that *within three years after having a stroke, 23 percent of individuals developed dementia.*

It is clear that the health of the vascular system is important for brain health and the prevention of Alzheimer's. Whether we are talking about the large arteries or the small micro-vessels, blood flow to the brain remains paramount to the health of each brain cell.

Finally, one day it happened. Mrs. Dell started out for the grocery store. It was four o'clock as usual. She turned left as she pulled out of the driveway and headed to a place she had gone almost daily for at least fifteen years. She knew the owner of the family store. She knew his wife by first name. She even asked the manager of the meat department located at the back of the one-room store how each of his children was doing.

That day Mrs. Dell drove the seven miles down the highway and simply passed the grocery store located on the left side of the road. Three traffic lights later, she crossed the river bridge. It wasn't until she stopped at the traffic light just past the bridge that she realized she knew exactly where she was, but she did not know why she was there. On the far corner was a restaurant with a parking lot big enough for her to turn around in so she could head back home. When Mr. Dell arrived home at his usual time of 5:30 and realized she had not fixed anything for dinner, Mrs. Dell proceeded to tell him about the strange event that had happened to her that afternoon.

He didn't say anything to her, but he knew. He didn't want to admit the sad reality of what was happening. He didn't know where this road was going to lead, but he had to acknowledge that this new path they were on was only the beginning.

Silent Strokes and the Brain

Eighty-five percent of adults over the age of fifty have blockages within the arteries of their hearts without any symptoms. Two-thirds of the time, the initial symptom is a full-blown heart attack.

Other times, people have a blockage of a large artery, such as a carotid artery in the neck, that can lead to a decrease in blood flow to the brain. It is easy to visualize how the sudden blockage of such a large artery can lead to a massive stroke that results in paralysis or the inability to speak. For most people, a full-blown stroke is a wake-up call. They decide to change their lifestyle habits in order to protect the health of their arteries.

But what about the brain? Is the same disease building up in the walls of the arteries of the brain without any symptoms showing? When micro-vessels are involved and the blood flow is markedly reduced to only a small area in the brain, a massive stroke does not occur. Instead, the person experiences a transient ischemic attack, a TIA, in which the symptoms are very mild and short-lived. In minutes, the person is "back to normal" as if nothing happened. They may be walking down the hall with a glass of water in their hand and all of a sudden drop the glass because they can't grasp it. Or they may begin to fall forward but catch themselves before hitting the floor. They wonder what happened and after going to the doctor are told they had a transient stroke. The stroke may be small, but it does result in the death of the portion of brain cells the artery was supplying. Studies show that these small injuries to the brain occur in one-third to one-half of older people.

Sometimes blockages in the micro-arteries cause silent strokes that people never know occurred. With a silent stroke, the warning bell and the blinking light don't go off. But the process continues. The silent damage continues in the micro-arteries, and more and more silent strokes occur. The only way one could know this is going on in their brain is through images of the brain that show the resulting scarring caused by multiple such incidents. And all the while, the result is damage to the barriers that are supposed to protect and control what is exchanged between the blood and the neuron network of the brain. As the blood-brain barriers are damaged, beta-amyloid continues to build up in the neurons of those areas.

The hippocampus is the part of the brain that affects memory the most. To emphasize the importance of keeping your arteries healthy by eating healthy, exercising, and keeping your goal weight, consider this statement from an article in the *Annals of Internal Medicine*. It's just a reminder, but I want to emphasize the association between the health of your arteries and the hippocampus. The statement reads, "Our results might be explained by the recent interesting finding that *the area of the brain most susceptible to ischemic damage, the hippocampus, is also one of the earliest areas of the brain to be affected by Alzheimer disease.*" This statement is one you should reread and concentrate on. From a medical standpoint, ischemic damage means that part of the brain is damaged by less blood flow to the area because the arteries are not healthy. The point being made is that memory problems are usually the initial symptoms of Alzheimer's. Such problems originate in the hippocampus, and that part of the brain is one of the earliest areas affected when there is a decrease in blood flow.

To understand how Alzheimer's develops, let's look at the two tiers of the mechanism of blood flow supplying the individual neurons within the brain.

First, we'll consider the heart and the larger arteries the heart utilizes to pump blood to the brain. I won't ask you to learn a lot of medical words, but one term I'd like you to know concerns plaque in the main arteries leading to the brain: *atherosclerosis*. Research shows a strong association between atherosclerosis and Alzheimer's. Most of the studies centered on the stiffness and thickness and plaques in the carotid arteries.

The other word I want you to remember deals with the smaller arteries within the substance of the brain, and disease of these smaller arteries is called *cerebrovascular disease*. "Cerebro" pertains to the brain and "vascular" pertains to the arteries. Disease of the arteries in three areas of the body can have an effect on Alzheimer's.

1. Disease of the arteries of the heart, which affects the pumping action of the heart muscle.
2. Disease in the arteries that feed the brain, the larger carotid arteries in the neck being the ones that are tested the most in evaluating the health of the arteries feeding your brain.
3. The smaller arteries within the brain.

Whether we are talking about the large arteries or the small micro-vessels, blood flow to the brain remains paramount in the health of each brain cell. An article in *Alzheimer's and Dementia* points out that in studies of blood flow in combination with beta-amyloid deposits, decreased blood flow has been observed before beta-amyloid deposition in individuals with Alzheimer's and has been proposed to contribute directly to the cognitive symptoms. The report also points out that some studies suggest the changes in the health of the arteries affect the clearance of beta-amyloid from the brain, which allows excess beta-amyloid to accumulate, resulting in the acceleration of the progression of Alzheimer's.

In a study of individuals followed by mental testing as well as brain MRI studies, researchers reported in the *New England Journal of Medicine*, "The presence of silent strokes at base line more than doubled the risk of dementia" as the patients were followed. Their conclusion: "Elderly people with silent strokes have an increased risk of dementia and a steeper decline in cognitive function than those without" such findings of silent strokes, meaning silent strokes cause dementia to worsen more rapidly. Basically, stage 1 individuals will progress more rapidly to stage 2, and stage 2 individuals will progress to stage 3 at a quicker pace.

You claim you've never had a stroke? That may be true, but if your arteries are damaged, you may have had a silent stroke and not know it. An article in the journal *Neurology* looked at autopsy cases in which over half of strokes found in the brain were silent. If someone had multiple such strokes, the odds for developing dementia were 2.67 times greater.

An article from the American Neurological Association reported on a study looking at the correlation between beta-amyloid plaques and damage to the brain caused by arterial problems that resulted in detectable mini-stroke changes within the brain. The conclusion was that older persons without any symptoms of Alzheimer's can have "considerable amounts" of beta-amyloid plaque. But here is the significant finding: *there was a fourfold increase in the odds of a person developing symptomatic dementia if they had arterial problems in addition to beta-amyloid depositions.* Arterial disease can lower the threshold for the symptoms of Alzheimer's to develop. Researchers concluded that small, silent strokes, as a result of reduced blood flow to the brain, increase the odds of dementia and lower memory function.

For the third time Mr. Dell asked me if I could help take away Mrs. Dell's car keys. The week before had proven to him that Mrs. Dell could not continue to drive. He was afraid she was going to run into something or not stop at a red light or a stop sign. He was afraid to let her drive even when he was in the car. He began his plea with a convincing statement: "Every time I say something to her about driving, she lashes out at me. It's not like her at all."

Mr. Dell had mentioned this to me twice before, but whenever I talked to her about it, her reaction was only a degree or two below anger. I decided it was time for a new plan of action.

"I'll talk with her doctor and explain my plan to him. You make her an appointment and take her to the doctor's office. You won't have to say anything. The doctor will take care of it all. I promise," I explained to Mr. Dell.

At the office visit, her doctor made a simple, straightforward statement about why Mrs. Dell should not be driving anymore. Then he pulled out his prescription pad and wrote a few words on it. He handed it to Mr. Dell. "This is a prescription reminder for her not to drive. Just show it to her anytime there is a question about driving."

The most surprising part of the visit was that Mrs. Dell accepted the directive from the doctor at face value. She did not utter one word of complaint or resistance as they left the doctor's office. Mr. Dell drove home and then did the one thing I instructed him to do. He went straight to the refrigerator and attached the prescription to the door. The note read just as I had asked the doctor to write it: *Mrs. Dell—No driving.*

"It's just a reminder," Mr. Dell told her.

Mr. Dell told me later that he couldn't count how many times she wanted to drive. Each time he took her to the refrigerator and pointed to the doctor's prescription. Each time she simply relented and asked him if he would drive her where she wanted to go. Soon she stopped asking where the car keys were.

By this time, she couldn't keep up with her bank statements. Mr. Dell would eventually take over paying the bills. And the sad part was that the day would come when Mrs. Dell would become bedridden. There would be no returning to things being normal again. She would have too much beta-amyloid gelling around her brain cells. Too many of them would have died.

Although she didn't know about lifestyle changes that could help her, I knew the reality of what was to come—she had just crossed over the finishing line of independence.

The time had come to select a caregiver to begin the journey with Mrs. Dell.

Can the Testing of Arteries Predict Dementia?

Take a step back to problems in a large artery that can lead to a massive stroke. Before such a stroke occurs, a disease process is taking place in the artery. There are no signs of a massive stroke, but something is beginning to cause the walls of the artery to become hard and thick. It is a silent process.

A report in the journal *Stroke* studied individuals who had no symptoms of stage 2 MCI or Alzheimer's dementia. You recall that in stage 1 of Alzheimer's, which is the stage before any symptoms show, there is evidence that beta-amyloid is developing in different areas of the brain, especially in the hippocampus, which affects memory to a large extent. This particular study utilized the same reasoning about the large carotid arteries feeding the brain. Can these arteries be tested to determine whether something is happening within the walls that will signal a greater risk for dementia down the road, before a stroke or any other symptom has occurred?

The primary factor in this study was the thickness of the walls of the carotid arteries. Previous studies had shown that carotid wall thickening is a measure of arterial disease that is happening before symptoms appear. Such thickening is seen prior to the problems of chest pain, heart attacks, or death from heart attacks and strokes. The question this study explored was whether this same early sign of arterial thickening offers any prediction concerning dementia. Do the early findings of thickness in carotid artery walls lead to Alzheimer's later on?

We know that thickening of the carotid arteries decreases blood flow to the brain to a degree, but the researchers wanted to determine if this was a risk factor for what was to come years down the road. Does a reduction of full blood flow to the neurons of the brain have an effect on mental reasoning and memory?

Researchers studied individuals who had no symptoms of diseased arteries in their hearts or brains. The thickness of their carotid artery walls was measured, and they underwent routine mental testing for dementia. These people were retested up to eight times over the following eleven years.

The results revealed that *those with greater thickness in the walls of their carotid arteries experienced a greater decline in their cognitive performance of memory and reasoning.* Their mental test scores were worse.

This report sounded an alarm for me as a surgeon who removed plaque from carotid arteries after someone experienced a stroke. It made me realize that the disease of the larger arteries I had operated on for years could eventually lead to a decline in mental awareness without the person knowing anything was happening. Even if you are not a surgeon, I hope this report sounds an alarm for you as well. Another article on silent strokes was published in the *New England Journal of Medicine*. In this study, researchers stated, "The presence of silent strokes more than doubled the risk of dementia." They went on to point out that people with silent strokes not only have an increased risk of dementia but also "a steeper decline in cognitive function" than those without silent strokes. Not only do silent strokes cause more Alzheimer's but they also cause dementia to worsen more rapidly. Basically, stage 1 individuals will progress more rapidly to stage 2, and stage 2 individuals will progress to stage 3 at a quicker pace.

Don't think it can't be happening to you. Even if you have no symptoms of disease in your arteries, the process may have begun. The takeaway of this report? Improve your arterial health now before symptoms appear later.

A report in the *American Journal of Geriatric Pharmacotherapy* gives these eye-opening statistics about the health of your arteries:

If you have had a stroke, you are three and a half to six times more likely to develop Alzheimer's.

If you have high blood pressure in midlife, you have four times the risk of developing Alzheimer's.

If you have diabetes, you have doubled your chance of developing Alzheimer's.

If you are obese in midlife, you have an increased risk of Alzheimer's in later life.

If you regularly exercise, you can reduce your risk of developing Alzheimer's.

If you regularly exercise even after symptoms of Alzheimer's have begun, even if you are over sixty-five years of age, you may prevent the decline of the mental process.

The takeaway from this article is that it's important to develop the lifestyles that protect the arteries in your brain as well as your heart by committing to develop personal lifestyle habits that ensure the proper health of your arteries.

Prevention supersedes any treatment known for Alzheimer's.

The enemy had been fairly silent. But I knew what was ahead—next week, next month, next year. It was coming like a freight train.

Mrs. Dell didn't always notice the effects of her disease, but *it cripples long before it kills*. I knew that. She didn't.

Overall, Mr. Dell handled the Alzheimer's situation well. He wasn't ready to end the dance—just yet. He didn't talk about it, and he stopped asking me about the future. He already knew—somewhat. He retired from real estate. His new job at the county courthouse made it possible for him to keep working but also being the best husband he could be. He knew they would need help someday, but he preferred to keep an eye on her for now.

He remained a good husband. As far as I knew, they never discussed her problem or where it was going to take her. He never worried about how it would affect him or how it would affect the two of them. He was committed. They still had quite a bit of distance to travel on the road ahead, and he would cover it with her and support her.

"I still love her," he told me. "And always will."

I knew he meant every word.

Vascular Risk Factors and Alzheimer's

Anything that causes damage to the arteries puts the arteries at risk. Each such factor is called a vascular risk factor. You want to avoid each of these risks. If you have a risk factor, you want to do something to remove that risk. The main risk factors that damage the arteries are high cholesterol, a sedentary lifestyle, excess weight, high blood pressure, and diabetes. More and more, the term *vascular risk factors* comes up when studying the causes of dementia.

An accumulation of beta-amyloid plaques is the hallmark diagnosis of Alzheimer's. However, some autopsies have revealed beta-amyloid plaques in people who didn't have any symptoms of Alzheimer's. Obviously, there is more to the disease. A report from the Alzheimer's Association gave this important assessment about the role of arteries and blood flow in helping to prevent the development of Alzheimer's: "Some autopsy studies suggest that plaques and tangles may be present in the brain without causing symptoms of cognitive decline *unless* the brain also shows evidence of vascular disease."

This statement gives us the most important insight into what could be a significant underlying cause of Alzheimer's and gives us hope that something can be done to prevent symptoms by protecting the health of the arteries. No one knows exactly how or why the beta-amyloid plaques form or the tau tangles develop, but we do know the risk factors that cause disease in the arteries, and we know how to control those risks. The article from the Alzheimer's Association went on to discuss how controlling the risk factors that affect the health of the arteries can reduce the chances of Alzheimer's dramatically. It also points out that most of these arterial risk factors of high cholesterol, being overweight, not exercising, diabetes, and high blood pressure are interrelated and connected to a general overall unhealthy lifestyle. Minimizing these risk factors even reduces the chance of developing certain common cancers.

We need to address these intertwined lifestyles simultaneously. I especially like their conclusion, which they put in bold print: "The public should know what the science concludes: certain healthy behaviors known to be effective for diabetes, cardiovascular disease, and cancer are also good for the brain health and for reducing the risk of cognitive decline."

This book is about identifying the risk factors and showing you how to control them. It is time we all realize our only hope for defeating Alzheimer's is prevention.

The vascular problem is caused by inflammation and blockage of your arteries. It affects the blood flow to each cell of your brain. The inflammation and blockage of your arteries may reside in your larger vessels, as in your carotid arteries, which you can feel on each side of your windpipe, or problems with smaller arteries that directly feed the oxygen and nutrients to those neurons in your brain. An article in the medical journal *Experimental Gerontology* reviewed a combination of reports looking at Alzheimer's and the health of the arteries. The article showed (1) arterial disease that affects both the arteries of the heart and the ones leading to the brain is associated with a higher prevalence of dementia; (2) an increased thickening of both large and small arteries feeding the brain is shown to cause an increased risk of dementia; (3) Alzheimer's disease patients have more disease in a group of arteries within the brain called the Circle of Willis, which feeds blood to both sides of the brain whenever one side is compromised; (4) individuals with a history of arterial disease resulting in a stroke have a higher prevalence of poor cognitive performance than those without a history of stroke; (5) generalized diseases in the arterial system are associated with a steeper decline in mental test scores; and (6) there is an increased risk for dementia in individuals who have signs of silent strokes, which can be found only on MRI studies of the brain.

Their summary statement on the importance of the health of the arteries in causing or protecting against Alzheimer's was this: *there is strong evidence that the presence of disease of the arteries is associated with an increased risk of cognitive impairment at all ages.*

Having one risk factor is bad enough, but what if you have more than one? Here is what the Finnish Cardiovascular Risk Factors, Aging, and Incidence of Dementia study showed concerning people who had more than one vascular risk factor. Researchers devised a unique set of risk scores for middle-aged people who had certain conditions that affected their arteries. They used these risk scores to predict the development of dementia twenty years later. Their prediction was based on the negative cardiovascular factors caused by disease of the arteries of the heart. The risk factors included high cholesterol, obesity, high blood pressure, and physical inactivity.

They found that the risk of Alzheimer's increased when a person had any one of the vascular risk factors mentioned. But they also found that the risk of Alzheimer's increased as the number of risk factors increased.

An article in the medical journal *Neurology* examined the multiple risk factors that are the basis for disease of the arteries. Researchers studied 1,138 elderly individuals who had no symptoms of Alzheimer's when the study began. They followed them in relation to which ones had certain lifestyles that are known risk factors for arterial disease. The risk factors they followed included heart disease and strokes caused by blockage and inflammation of the arteries of the heart, high blood pressure, diabetes, and smoking.

All of these were related to risk to the health of the arteries of these individuals. Whenever heart disease is mentioned, one has to relate that to LDL cholesterol, which is the main culprit in disease in the arteries of the heart. One important factor they pointed out concerning how heart disease is related to Alzheimer's was, there is a higher frequency of beta-amyloid plaque among people with arterial disease in their heart compared with individuals of similar age who did not have heart disease.

The researchers concluded that arterial risk factors are very seldom isolated. In other words, those who are overweight usually do not eat properly nor do the majority of them exercise. Heart disease, increased cholesterol, increased blood pressure, diabetes, smoking, as well as being overweight or obese are all related to Alzheimer's.

This study also concluded that *the risk of Alzheimer's increased with the number of vascular risk factors.* Do you have any of the vascular risk factors? Do you have more than one? Or two? Or three?

One statistic concerning these risk factors offers hope that we can avoid developing Alzheimer's. It was stated in a recent study in Europe called the Prevention of Dementia by Intensive Vascular Care study. Researchers found that *87 percent of the study participants had at least one modifiable risk factor.* None of us live the perfect life for the prevention of Alzheimer's. But we can learn the risk factors we possess and begin making lifestyle changes.

If you are like me, when one person tells me something that makes sense, I usually remember it for a little while. If two or three other people tell me something similar, I pay more attention. After hearing the same information a number of times, I commit to changing my original thinking. I hope these studies convince you that whether we are talking about stage 1, 2, or 3, the health of the arteries is of utmost importance in the fight against Alzheimer's.

Shortly after Mrs. Dell's doctor visit when she received her no-driving prescription, Mr. Dell shared an interesting observation with me. Mrs. Dell began wearing jewelry she hadn't worn in years. Mr. Dell explained, "She smiles every time anyone compliments the jewelry, and her response is always the same: 'I haven't worn it in years. Do you like it?' She says that every time."

I wondered, *Is she considering the reality that now is the time to enjoy all she has?* I think Mrs. Dell realized something important for all of us. Today is the day to live life to its fullest. Take a moment to be thankful for today.

What If You Already Have Symptoms?

An article in the medical journal *Neurology* detailed a study presented at the International Conference on Prevention of Dementia. This article helps us understand why we should be doing everything possible to reduce each risk factor, even if the symptoms of Alzheimer's have appeared, even if we just visited the doctor and were told we probably have Alzheimer's disease.

This study was performed on individuals who had been diagnosed with Alzheimer's. Researchers pinpointed several of the vascular risk factors these people had to see if treatment helped to slow the mental decline normally seen in Alzheimer's. Ninety-three percent of the people had one or more of the vascular risk factors. Researchers found that treatment of these factors resulted in a slower decline as shown on follow-up mental tests.

When the arteries of the heart are damaged by the LDL cholesterol and inflammation resulting in decreased blood flow to the muscles of the heart, the muscles can cause a pain in the chest when they are not getting enough oxygen to function as necessary. This may be on exertion or when the muscle is stressed to pump more blood. This pain is called angina. The study noted that angina was associated with a more rapid mental decline once Alzheimer's was diagnosed. This study listed the arterial risk factors that caused the heart disease of angina to develop. Included were high cholesterol, diabetes, high blood pressure, and the presence of atherosclerosis, which you recall is the buildup of plaque in the larger arteries of the body. All of the factors that cause angina have been associated with an increased risk of Alzheimer's.

The two key groups that benefited the most from treatment were those with high cholesterol and those who already had disease in their arteries.

This study showed that the more disease a person has in their arteries, the faster Alzheimer's symptoms develop and the worse they become. But this particular study also showed that even if a person has symptoms of Alzheimer's, it is never too late for them to change their lifestyle habits to slow the process. I like the title they gave this study: "Treatment of Vascular Risk Factors Is Associated with Slower Decline in Alzheimer's Disease."

Even in stages 2 and 3, we can fight the vascular risk factors with all our might.

I'll never forget the day Mr. Dell called with an excitement I had not heard from him in a long time. "I have such great news," is how he began. "I have just returned from the grocery store, where I ran into an old friend. She told me she knew about a very special caregiver named Katy. She knew we were looking for someone and that Katy was available. An elderly lady she'd been taking care of recently passed away." Mr. Dell continued, "My friend said that Katy was the one person she would want taking care of her if she ever needed such help. She said Katy would show love like a daughter would show a mother." He ended the one-way conversation with an exciting statement: "I knew in an instant Katy would be perfect for us. Katy is the one."

The Big Question

Deposits of beta-amyloid in the brain are a prerequisite for a diagnosis of Alzheimer's. Even if you don't have symptoms, the destructive process of Alzheimer's has begun. Even though there are no medications as of yet that prevent or cure Alzheimer's, many trials are going on in an attempt to find a drug to slow or halt the progress of the disease. Right now some of the main goals of drug treatment center on getting rid of the beta-amyloid plaques. What we don't know is this: even if we are able to dissolve the beta-amyloid plaques, will doing so cure the disease?

No one knows that answer. Not drug companies. Not medical researchers. Nobody knows at this time. The underlying question is whether beta-amyloid is the cause of the disease or simply a by-product of the disease process. Could there be a battle going on elsewhere, and the beta-amyloid plaques are just dead soldiers lying on the ground? If we remove these dying and dead soldiers, can we win the war? Is beta-amyloid the problem or the result of the problem? Could disease in the blood-brain barriers of the arterial system be where the battlefield really is?

The removal of excess beta-amyloid from the brain is of pivotal importance for the regulation of beta-amyloid levels in the brain. Anything that impedes this regulation contributes to greater beta-amyloid levels in the brain. A high percentage of Alzheimer's patients show damage in the micro-arterial network of the blood-brain barriers.

If we decide to fight Alzheimer's, where do we attack? The beta-amyloid plaques or the blood-brain barriers? Or the large carotid arteries? Or the arteries in the heart? Or is the battlefield somewhere else we don't even know about? Is there more than one battlefield?

These are all questions researchers are asking in an attempt to locate where to fire their cannons. Several drug trials have come up empty-handed. What we do know about decreasing our chances of developing Alzheimer's involves lifestyle habits we can and should control. It is beyond me why anyone who wants to do all they can to lower their odds of developing Alzheimer's would hope for and wait on a possible drug that may or may not help. There are things we can do right now that can help. Right now the only possible cure is prevention.

Remember this statement: *the aging process is dependent on the health of the arteries.* The key to such health lies within lifestyle factors we can learn to control.

We didn't know about these risk factors back then, but if Mrs. Dell were to go to the doctor today, she would likely be instructed differently. She would be placed on the medication, but her doctor also would have explained the risk factors she should be working on to slow the progression of the disease. Her doctor would have told her that the factors causing disease of her arteries have an impact on the progression of Alzheimer's.

She would have gotten information on things she could do to protect every artery supplying every nerve cell in order to get the oxygen and nutrients to each neuron and to every synapse that came out of that neuron.

Potentially, she would learn the difference between the good fats and the bad fats. I would like to believe the next time she went to the grocery store, she would look at the nutrition fact box to see if what she was buying included any saturated fat. She would know the bad fats were found in red meats and dairy products like cheese, butter, and cream. She would quit eating her usual pint of ice cream every night and give up her ice cream bars.

Not only would Mrs. Dell know by heart which bad fats to avoid but she would also know what the good fats are. She would cook Mr. Dell vegetables every evening and serve him the monounsaturated and polyunsaturated fats in salmon, nuts, and olive oil. She would know that she ought to substitute the good fats for the bad rather than stopping the bad fats and substituting the high sugar foods in their place. No more donuts, pastries, and cakes for dessert. She would begin to understand how important fiber is to her diet. She would fix a breakfast of oatmeal or a high-fiber cereal with three fruits to finish out the meal. And the more fruit she could get into her bowl, the better. She would incorporate more peas and legumes and nuts, and her cooking oils would change from animal fat to olive oil or canola oil.

Since Mrs. Dell was "pudgy," as she called herself, she would eat fruits and vegetables and fiber that would include fewer calories. She would even explain to Mr. Dell that fruits and vegetables give them the most food for the least calories. She would eliminate all her snacks until she reached her ideal weight.

Plus, rather than spending most of the day tending her flower garden, she would devote thirty minutes, six days a week, to exercising. She might have bought a treadmill or joined the local gym.

I would like to believe today's world would be a different place for Mrs. Dell and her war with Alzheimer's. I want to encourage you, before it's too late, to review the paragraphs above and commit to making changes.

Honestly, I don't know whether Mrs. Dell would have done all of the above. I would like to believe she would.

The dilemma I continued to face was how much to tell Mrs. Dell. As a doctor, I realized there were things she probably was not aware of. How much should she know?

Mr. Dell said not to tell her too much. He asked that I wait and let her ask whatever she wanted to know. He didn't want me to say anything that would be anxiety-provoking to her. "I want her to know I will always be here for her," he closed our discussion. As hard as it was for me to agree, I made the decision to honor his request.

5

Midlife and Alzheimer's

Katy spoke with some trepidation. "I want to tell you something." She said it like she was going to be a tattletale. "I know you would want to know this. Mrs. Dell has quit making her favorite cookies. You know, the ones she always filled the cookie jar with. She doesn't make them anymore."

Every time I visited, Katy had a new detail to tell me. I explained to her that this was simply the early stages of Mrs. Dell's Alzheimer's. There would be more and more events she would notice. I then encouraged her to keep Mrs. Dell comfortable and to help her carry on her life day by day as normally as possible. Katy's job was difficult, having to experience the everyday debilitating changes that accompanied this dreadful disease.

"I knew something was wrong. Two batches ago, she forgot the chocolate, and the last batch she made . . ." Katy paused. "Had too much sugar in it."

It wasn't long before my next visit. Katy reported, "She couldn't find her credit card. We all looked everywhere. She checked her pocketbook three times, searched under everything on the kitchen counter, went in her bedroom to check the bedside table, and looked in her pocketbook one more time. She couldn't find it. Two days later, she was looking through a magazine beside her easy chair. She let out a shout. 'I found it.'"

In early reports about Alzheimer's, the people studied were in their later years and had already developed Alzheimer's. As a result, some of these people did not seem to have the risk factors that we now know lead to the disease. For example, their blood pressure at eighty years of age was low, or they were skinny, or their cholesterol was normal. At this late stage of life, risk factors may all be on the low end rather than the high.

An article in the journal *Vascular Health and Risk Management* noted that as we age, certain numbers relating to the risk factors for Alzheimer's begin changing. During later years, total cholesterol decreases, perhaps because of a change in diet and nutrition. Blood pressure and body weight also begin to decline. Because of these changes, studying someone's cholesterol and weight and blood pressure in later life distorts the findings in relation to Alzheimer's. Mrs. Dell was overweight, being what she called plump in midlife, but as her Alzheimer's progressed, she became less and less so, ending up in the skinny column. In later life, her cholesterol was not high, partially because no one brought her any ice cream bars or other bad foods available to her in midlife.

When studying Alzheimer's, what is important to note is what people were like in midlife.

It was evening, and Mrs. Dell was finishing a more active day than usual. Mr. Dell was attending a dinner meeting. Mrs. Dell and I sat for a while saying nothing; I reached for and gently held her hand. She closed her eyes and relaxed her head on the back of the sofa. It was the fall of the year, my favorite season. I thought about two days earlier when I had ridden my motorcycle on the Blue Ridge Parkway in North Carolina. It was peak autumn season, and the leaves were beautiful as they fell from the trees. Right in the middle of my ride, a gust of wind blew a bunch of bright orange and yellow leaves right in front of me. There were so many leaves that they almost blocked my vision.

I looked over at Mrs. Dell, and out of the blue, I recalled the first verse of a Henry Wadsworth Longfellow poem I had learned in fifth grade. I hadn't thought of that verse about autumn since grammar school.

> The day is cold, and dark, and dreary;
> It rains, and the wind is ever weary;
> The vine still clings to the moldering wall,
> But at each gust the dead leaves fall.

I looked at Mrs. Dell's relaxed face. She was asleep. It was such a pleasant sight. I let go my grip on her relaxed hand and placed both of my hands into my lap. The picture of Mrs. Dell became so clear. The season was beautiful, but I knew the harsh winter was on its way. And it kept running through my mind as I looked at her—at each gust, the dead leaves are falling.

Vascular Risk Factors and Midlife

In recent years, researchers have begun going back in patients' records to examine whether patients with certain medical conditions in midlife were more likely to develop Alzheimer's than those without such conditions. Such studies showed that the medical condition of someone in their forties and fifties was very predictive of whether they would develop Alzheimer's dementia in their later years. These studies were also able to determine which factors made people more prone to Alzheimer's.

People who had the five vascular risk factors—high cholesterol, high blood pressure, diabetes, excess weight, or a sedentary lifestyle—in midlife were found to have a higher incidence of Alzheimer's than those who exercised, ate properly to keep their cholesterol low, and were at an ideal weight, which was also associated with not having diabetes or high blood pressure.

A basic study was done through the University of Kuopio in Finland. Over nine thousand people were tested for total cholesterol during midlife and followed to see how significant elevated cholesterol was for increasing their risk of

Alzheimer's. Doctors encourage patients to aim for a total cholesterol of under 200. *Researchers found that someone whose total cholesterol was over 240 during midlife increased their risk for Alzheimer's disease in later life by 66 percent.* Some numbers reported in the journal *Obesity* explain that what a person weighs in midlife correlates with whether they have a greater risk of developing Alzheimer's in later life. This report examined sixteen medical studies that evaluated the relationship between BMI and Alzheimer's. BMI, body mass index, is a weight-to-height ratio frequently used in medical studies concerning a person's weight. Normal is considered 20 to 25, overweight is 25 to 30, and obese is over 30. These numbers are not exact. Just because a person is in the normal category doesn't necessarily mean they are at their ideal weight. Nevertheless, most research studies utilize BMI. The result of this study showed that *women who were obese in midlife had a 3.08 times greater risk of developing Alzheimer's. The increased risk for men was 2.45 times greater.* The study's takeaway thought was this: having a normal BMI in midlife equates with the lowest risk of dementia, while an obese BMI in midlife causes the greatest risk.

An article in the medical journal *Brain* pointed out that a decreased fitness of the heart in midlife was associated with an increased risk of early-onset stage 2 MCI as well as stage 3 Alzheimer's dementia later in life.

I use this example to stress that even if you aren't old enough to be concerned about Alzheimer's, you should begin in midlife and even before to fight the aging process.

By now Katy and Mrs. Dell were the best of friends. They were together around the clock. I knew Katy hated to see any negative changes in Mrs. Dell's behavior. I think Katy equated her excellent care of Mrs. Dell with an eventual improvement or at least a lack of decline. But on this particular visit, Katy shared a change she had noticed over the past several weeks.

"Every evening we watch the news and then *Jeopardy*. About four months ago, I began noticing that when a contestant got an answer right, I clapped and smiled and said, 'That's great.' But she just looked at me. She used to clap, but she just looked at me. It was like she didn't understand what they were doing.

"I still turn it on for her—every night because I know she likes it—but she doesn't watch it like she used to."

Katy didn't want to see Mrs. Dell slide. Neither did I. I realized her yesterdays were disappearing and her tomorrows were becoming more and more uncertain. A strange thought ran through my head: *her leaves were not yet dead, but the colors were beginning to change.*

In those days, we didn't have MRIs or PET scans to measure the progression of buildup of the beta-amyloid in Mrs. Dell's brain. But Mr. Dell's awareness was almost as good as any medical testing. His observations were similar to what medical journals today report. Recent memory is one of the first to go in the hippocampus, and if an MRI and PET scan were done, there would be images of the beta-amyloid in that part of the brain, as well as a decrease in the volume of that area because of the shrinkage caused by the dead cells. The same reports would be made if an autopsy were performed on such a brain at that particular stage of Alzheimer's.

The only indicator I had, at the time, was Mr. Dell's reports. It was one of the first "recent memory" problems he had given me in a long time. He was learning to live with them, but his sadness was increasingly evident.

"She was supposed to pick up dessert for the supper club. She forgot."

Lifestyle Changes

Let's take a quick look at some of the lifestyle changes that help you in the prevention of Alzheimer's no matter what age range you may presently be in. What does the medical literature reveal about such lifestyle changes in general in relation to Alzheimer's? Are certain lifestyles found more often in people who have Alzheimer's versus individuals who do not have such dementia? It is pretty simple to look at the literature and realize that people who have Alzheimer's fit into certain categories and those who don't have it fit into a different grouping. As you read, you will see that the people who now have Alzheimer's were overweight in midlife, or had high LDL cholesterol, or were inactive. You can decide that you want to avoid those unhealthy lifestyle choices, especially when you realize that those without such medical problems have far less chance of developing Alzheimer's.

Reports in some of the leading medical journals offer these insights into how our lifestyles, especially in midlife, affect whether we develop Alzheimer's in later life or not. A variety of specific studies published in the journals *Lancet Neurology*, the *Annals of Internal Medicine*, *Neurology*, and the *Archives of Neurology* all point out that your chances for having Alzheimer's in later life are greater if in midlife your blood pressure is elevated or your BMI is elevated. That means being overweight or obese is not good. Also, your chances are worse if your LDL cholesterol is elevated during your midlife years. Diabetes is associated with an increased risk of Alzheimer's throughout life, but the association is even stronger when it occurs in midlife. You want to begin the battle as young as you can.

One such study published in the journal *Neurology* emphasizes the importance of beginning the defeat of Alzheimer's as early as possible, even during the early years of midlife. It described how artery risk factors in midlife relate to the risk of Alzheimer's in late life.

The investigation began by studying over eight thousand participants who were between the ages of forty and forty-four. Their medical records were evaluated thirty years later to determine who developed dementia. Then, these participants' midlife medical records were reexamined and correlated to see if those who had arterial risk factors in their midlife period developed dementia in later life.

What they found was astonishing. They discovered that *"the presence of multiple cardiovascular (arterial) risk factors at midlife substantially increases risk of late-life dementia in a dose dependent manner.*" Significantly, they listed specific arterial risk factors—high cholesterol, high blood pressure, diabetes, and smoking—and stated that they were each associated with an increased risk of dementia in later life. The study reported the statistics by each risk factor:

High cholesterol—42 percent more likely to have dementia

Obesity—3.1 times more likely

Overweight—2 times more likely

High blood pressure—24 percent more likely

Diabetes—46 percent more likely

Smoking—26 percent more likely

Now, what about if you have more than one of the above going on in your body? Here are the numbers they found concerning the risks you are taking if you don't do anything about it.

One of the above—27 percent more likely to develop dementia

Two of the above—70 percent more likely

Three of the above—200 percent or two times more likely

Four of the above—237 percent more likely

Note that being obese is the worst of all, partly because so many other risk factors for your arteries are linked to being overweight.

Every item in the list is also a risk factor for disease of your arteries. This sounds a loud alarm on the significance the health of your arteries plays in Alzheimer's.

No one knows the exact cause of Alzheimer's. It is known that the more beta-amyloid builds up around the neurons in the brain and the more tau protein within those cells becomes tangled, the greater the symptoms. The above risk factors are associated with increased buildup of beta-amyloid. But what exactly causes the excess beta-amyloid? Is it the actual beta-amyloid that causes the problem, or is it something else that simply results in too much beta-amyloid in those particular locations? Normally, there is a certain amount of beta-amyloid produced and a certain amount of it removed into the bloodstream. Is too much beta-amyloid produced, or is there a blockage of the drainage process resulting in too much left in the brain?

There is an interesting article published in *Experimental Gerontology* about a study done in Austria that shines some light on this question. This study points out some possibilities. One being that the arterial risk factors of having high cholesterol, diabetes, and disease of the small arteries around the neurons may cause damage to the cerebrovascular system, which could cause small strokes in the area. Or those same risk factors could cause a hindrance of the beta-amyloid clearance where it does not cross the blood-brain barrier where it gets back into the blood to be carried away. Such a disruption would result in an increase of beta-amyloid left remaining in the brain tissue.

I find this interesting in understanding why we need to develop our lifestyles to avoid such risk factors that may be causing the problem. This report is contemplating that if the risk factors mentioned above are causing this problem at the interchange of giving the brain the good nutrients and carrying away the excess waste products, then this could be the initial step of a cascade of events that may make matters worse, such as an inflammatory response in the area as well as oxidation, which could affect the tau protein. The scenario begins with the arterial problems and ends with there being inflammation and oxidation of the surrounding area, resulting in the degeneration of the neuron and the buildup of beta-amyloid.

This cascade from beginning to end involves beta-amyloid throughout. With arterial disease, the barrier that lets products *into* the neuron complex as well as the buildup waste products *out of* the arena malfunctions. As you recall, what researchers are describing is the blood-brain barrier previously mentioned.

In this study, researchers postulate that the accumulation of beta-amyloid in the brain is caused by the disease process going on at the blood-brain barrier, and this process results in an imbalance between the normal production of the beta-amyloid and the normal clearance of the product.

This report points out that because of all this dysfunction of the cerebrovascular workings in the area where the arteries interchange with the neurons, there can be a resulting breakdown of the blood-brain barrier. Such a breakdown could allow substances that are not supposed to be able to get through the barriers to get into the neuron areas, as well as not properly regulating substances that need to get out of the neuron areas. A little complicated to read, but whether we understand it completely or not, it makes us realize how complex Alzheimer's is, as well as how important the absolute health of our arteries is in combating the enemy. Again, the health of your arterial system is supreme.

Medicine versus Lifestyle Changes to Protect Your Arteries

There was another sad report in the news the other day. The headline stated, "Failed Study, Dimmed Hopes in Hunt for Alzheimer's Treatment." The article went on to say, "A treatment for Alzheimer's failed to slow mental decline in a widely anticipated study, ending hope that researchers had finally found a drug that does more to help those suffering from the fatal, mind-robbing disease." The next sentence showed what lost hope means, even to those who don't have the disorder. It read, "The pharmaceutical company's shares plunged Wednesday before markets opened."

Alzheimer's robs the mind. So we must continue looking at what we can do now instead of hoping for a pill that will help once we have the disease.

Your risk for developing Alzheimer's is 10 to 15 percent. Those are not very good odds. If you are sitting in a room with five or six other people, the odds are that one of you most likely will develop Alzheimer's. And nearly half of all people eighty-five and older will have Alzheimer's. You can't control the genes you were born with, but there are factors you can control. Some factors increase your chances of developing Alzheimer's, and some factors significantly decrease your chances. You want to begin doing all you can to eliminate the risk factors and making positive lifestyle choices as soon as possible. Parts 3 and 4 will help you do just that.

Morning had always been Mrs. Dell's favorite time of day. She and Mr. Dell would eat together, then he would leave for work. He would kiss her on the forehead and say good-bye. Every day she would respond with a smile and say, "I'll see you soon. I love you."

But now the time of day began to mean less and less to Mrs. Dell. She still ate breakfast most mornings, usually after Mr. Dell had left for work, after he had fixed his own cereal or toast with jelly. Mrs. Dell never cooked or fixed her own lunch anymore. Katy prepared something, then called her to come eat.

The change didn't seem to bother her. Soon she would be back working with her flowers, digging around the big rose bush and putting mulch in place. She spent all afternoon repeating the process three times on the same bush. But she still smiled if you asked if you could help her. Her life was beginning to become tangled concerning memory, time, and events. Tau tangles were increasing also. Her memory was beginning to fade. Alzheimer's was setting its deliberate, unhurried pace.

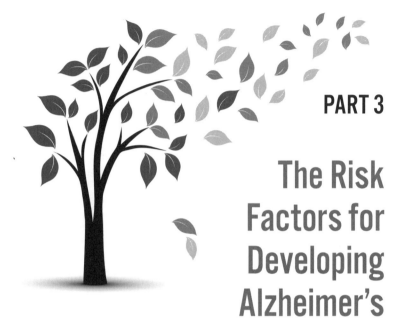

PART 3

The Risk Factors for Developing Alzheimer's

6

Your Course Determines
Your Destination

Research into modifiable lifestyle factors has changed our thinking about Alzheimer's. It is no longer seen as an untreatable and almost inevitable part of the aging process. It is now seen as potentially preventable. The National Institute on Aging and the Alzheimer's Association have recently stressed what they call the preclinical stage of Alzheimer's. These findings of the presymptomatic period of Alzheimer's have opened some exciting new horizons concerning prevention of the most dreaded disease we know. Yet most people do not realize that the risk of Alzheimer's can be reduced.

New ways to study the brain are being employed to evaluate the earlier stages of Alzheimer's. We can see and follow changes in the brain long before there are any symptoms. There is a lot of excitement about being able to diagnose the disease even before signs begin to show, because if there are any future therapies that are developed, Alzheimer's can be attacked before symptoms occur. We could begin medication before symptoms arrive, but the problem lies in the fact that there are no known drugs that can treat the process by preventing it or even slowing it down. Even though drug research is ongoing, there still is no treatment or cure.

The one misconception you must pay special attention to right now is that there is nothing you can do to help prevent Alzheimer's or to slow down the process. The truth is that how you live has a significant effect on the course of Alzheimer's. Some factors *increase* your chances of developing Alzheimer's. Some factors *decrease* your chances of developing Alzheimer's. Always remember: the course you are on determines your destination.

The next five chapters focus on the risk factors that increase your chances of developing Alzheimer's.

I believe you will eat differently because you learned that certain foods increase your chances of developing Alzheimer's and eating other foods reduces your chances.

I think you will look at exercise in a completely different light. Only one in four people over fifty exercise, and most people do not realize that physical activity can affect Alzheimer's as well as heart disease and even some cancers.

The more you realize how being overweight and obese affects your brain, the more you will consider the impact your lifestyle has on your future, as well as that of your spouse and children. Lifestyle is a hundredfold more significant than any medicine in the case of Alzheimer's.

The Five Risk Factors

An article in the journal *Neurology* discussed these risk factors. Researchers studied individuals who had Alzheimer's and found that *93 percent of them had at least one risk factor, and these risk factors are preventable.* Even if the patients had symptoms, if their risk factors were corrected, there was a slower progression of the disease and reasoning loss. This study showed it is never too late to aggressively defeat the factors that cause the disease to progress.

The vascular risk factors that have a detrimental effect on the health of the arteries are also the risk factors for Alzheimer's. They all affect the arteries that supply blood to the brain, therefore affecting whether the brain is receiving the essentials it needs to carry on normal mental function. The five factors that increase the risk of Alzheimer's are:

1. High cholesterol
2. A sedentary lifestyle
3. Excess weight
4. High blood pressure
5. Diabetes

Each of these factors enhances your chances of developing Alzheimer's, but the more of these risk factors you have, the greater your risk of developing Alzheimer's and the stronger your motivation should be to make changes in how you live.

Mrs. Dell fit into the category of not doing something to defeat her risk factors. If she had known, she might have committed to living differently. She might have changed her diet and started an exercise routine. Before long she could have reached her ideal weight. But she didn't know, and she was enjoying life. For her, there was no reason to change.

She continued giving Mr. Dell a hug every time he surprised her with the box of ice cream bars she liked so much. She sometimes ate more than one at a sitting. What she didn't know was that multiple factors were causing her Alzheimer's to progress, day by day, down a road she didn't need to be traveling. Oh, how I wish there had been a different road for Mrs. Dell.

The Process Is Irreversible; Prevention Is Crucial

Finding a cure for Alzheimer's won't happen, because once brain cells die, they cannot be brought back to life. New cells may form, but the disease out-fights the number of new soldiers and wins the battle. The plaques and tangles—the hallmark of Alzheimer's—cause irreparable damage, and neurons perish. Nothing can bring brain cells back.

Alzheimer's is a progressive disease. Similar to when Mrs. Dell was diagnosed many years ago, there is still no medicine that can prevent or halt the inevitable declining process. Imprint on your mind one major fact that every doctor who treats with medicine and every surgeon who operates on disease knows: it is much more important to prevent than to treat. I operated on lung cancer and arteries my entire surgical career. I took lung cancers out of men and women who had spouses and children and grandchildren who depended on them. Most smoked a pack of cigarettes a day for many years. The overwhelming majority wished they had never smoked. In hindsight, most said, "If only I had known." Had they known, they never would have smoked. They would have done anything to prevent their cancer. Think about their examples as you consider Alzheimer's. Think about what you can do to lower your chances of developing it. Even if there is some medication that proves helpful in the future, just realize that once a cell dies, the symptoms can't be reversed. Medicine will never be as good as prevention. Learn and do all you can to make your risk as low as possible.

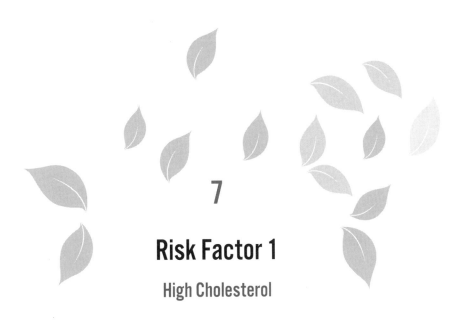

7

Risk Factor 1

High Cholesterol

We have a problem. Most of us do not know what is going on in our bodies. Damage happens unseen, and we have no idea that the choices we make are causing the damage. Most people don't realize that the health of the arteries determines the aging process.

Let me help you visualize why your cholesterol matters. Picture in your mind small particles floating around in your blood. Some of these particles are good; some are bad. The bad particles work their way through the lining of an artery and get into the wall itself. That area in the arterial wall becomes a miniature battlefield. The body pours in soldier-type cells and fluids in an attempt to get rid of the foreign invader. Over time this reaction can lead to either a rupture or plaque buildup in the affected artery. This is a silent process. It doesn't cause you any pain. It doesn't give you a headache or make your chest hurt. The battle goes on quietly while you order extra cheese on your hamburger and ask for extra cream sauce on your steak.

Damage to the arteries is one of the greatest problems we have in America and results in over half of the deaths every year due to heart attacks and strokes. We now know that the same arterial damage plays a significant role in Alzheimer's. We all need to know what cholesterol is doing within our bodies as we lead our everyday lives.

Let's learn more about cholesterol and how when we choose to protect ourselves against heart attacks and strokes we are also protecting ourselves against Alzheimer's. We are getting a two-for-one health bonus.

"So you think she's getting worse?" I asked Katy. She didn't answer. It was like she didn't want to answer. I could see the rain on the windows and the pine trees blowing. It was a terrible day outside.

"Yes," Katie finally answered. "I don't think you believe me, but I'm afraid she is."

Katy looked saddened as she looked me in the eye and said, "Two weeks ago, I found the checkbook lying open on the table. Three checks were written—one to the power company, one for county tax, and one for yard work. Mrs. Dell had signed her first name on one, but there was no signature on the other two. She had written the dollar amount in the proper place on all three checks but had not spelled out the amount on the second line like you're supposed to." Katy looked almost frightened. "All three showed who the checks were going to, but only the first two numbers of the zip code were written on each envelope. That was the last time I let her pay the bills."

Katy looked away but didn't move. It was like she had more to say but didn't want to go further. She picked up a dish towel and began walking past me toward the kitchen. All she said as she passed was, "And she can't find where the dishes are kept. She keeps putting them in the wrong cupboard."

What Is Cholesterol?

Cholesterol is a fatty substance that exists in the outer layer of every cell in the body, maintaining each cell's membrane. It is involved in the production of sex hormones as well as hormones released by the adrenal glands. It insulates nerve fibers. It is significant in the metabolism of certain vitamins, including A, D, and E. It is essential to the body.

Cholesterol is carried through the bloodstream combined with a protein. Cholesterol combined with a protein makes a molecule called a lipoprotein. There are two main types of lipoproteins. You will see them on your lab report as Low Density Lipoprotein cholesterol and High Density Lipoprotein cholesterol, or LDL and HDL. Here is an easy way to remember them. LDL is "lethal," and HDL is a "hero." You want your lethal number to be as low as possible and your hero number to be as high as possible.

Your cholesterol numbers are to your body what warning lights are to your car. If you don't know your cholesterol numbers, get a test done today to find out what they are. Then come back to this book to learn about the lifestyle choices that will put you in charge of your numbers. There are many things you can do to control your LDL cholesterol as well as your HDL cholesterol. Those numbers your doctor gives you don't just happen by chance.

Katy continued hoping that Mrs. Dell's medicine would cure her. Katy wanted her well. That's why she kept asking, "Is her medicine helping?"

I explained there was no medicine that would cure Alzheimer's nor slow the deposit of beta-amyloid nor decrease the appearance of the tau tangles. "Medicine may help the symptoms some, but it won't prevent what is going on in her brain. Maybe the medicine will help her feel better," I explained.

At first Katy didn't reply. Then she said slowly and thoughtfully, "Well, I always thought the earlier a doctor made the diagnosis of something, the sooner the patient could be put on medicine. I thought there would be more hope to cure it or at least slow it down until another new medicine comes along that can cure it. To me, it doesn't look like the medicine is slowing down the Alzheimer's, and I don't see that it's helping Mrs. Dell, but I am going to continue giving it to her because the doctor ordered it. I'm still hoping for a cure."

I decided it would be better if I didn't explain to Katy that whatever was already lost was lost for good. Any leaf that has fallen from the tree cannot be replaced on the limb.

Total Cholesterol, LDL Cholesterol, and HDL Cholesterol

Everybody has heard about cholesterol, but not everyone knows what it means. People tell me that their physician told them "it" is too high and they need some medication to get "it" down. That's about as far as their understanding goes.

To understand cholesterol, we need to understand three numbers:

1. Total cholesterol
2. LDL cholesterol
3. HDL cholesterol

There was concern on Katy's face. "About a month ago, Mrs. Dell started having trouble working the microwave. She would confuse seconds and minutes. She couldn't understand why it didn't work properly. After the third or fourth time, she would give up and quit and leave the popcorn or coffee in the microwave. One time I found her cup in the microwave, but the coffee had exploded all over the inside. I asked her how long she heated her coffee, and she said thirty seconds. I told her she must have hit thirty minutes. Two days later, she did it again."

"Tell you what we'll do," I responded to Katy. "We'll get a new microwave that has buttons that say 'coffee' and 'popcorn.' It's a lot easier that way."

Katy responded, "But she's never had trouble with the microwave before."

Total Cholesterol

When your doctor tells you your cholesterol is too high, they are usually talking about your total cholesterol number. Most patients don't realize that the total cholesterol is the sum of their bad LDL cholesterol and their good HDL cholesterol. There are some additional cholesterol particles within that total number, but they are fairly insignificant in understanding what is going on.

When a physician says your cholesterol is too high, what they are actually saying is that your lethal LDL cholesterol is too high. This is because your total cholesterol number is made up mostly of your LDL cholesterol, and if it is high, your total number will be high.

If you are told you must get your cholesterol down, your doctor means you should get your LDL cholesterol down. When your doctor says they are giving you a medication to lower your cholesterol, what they should say is that they are giving you a medication to lower your LDL cholesterol. Your doctor should then explain that the primary causes of high LDL cholesterol are eating the wrong foods that contain the bad fat, being overweight, and living a sedentary lifestyle.

The *Journal of the American Medical Association* published a study on the life expectancy of younger men who had a favorable total cholesterol level compared to men of the same age who had an unfavorable total cholesterol level. The conclusions should astound you. The men who had a favorable, lower level of total cholesterol had a life expectancy of 3.8 to 8.7 years longer than the ones with an unfavorable, higher level of total cholesterol. There was a continuous, proportional relationship between the amount of total cholesterol and the life expectancy difference. *Those who took their eating habits the most seriously had the additional 8.7 years.*

In the past, Mrs. Dell had routine blood tests that showed her total cholesterol was elevated. Her doctor didn't explain to her that most of that total number represented the lethal LDL cholesterol that would be responsible for the blockages in the arteries in her brain. Her physician knew high cholesterol was bad for her heart. Back then he wasn't aware that cholesterol was bad for her brain. He didn't explain the damage those ice cream bars were doing to her brain. He didn't know. Even if he had known and had tried to explain it to her, I'm not sure it would have registered with her.

Mrs. Dell was enjoying life to its fullest. At that time in her life, neither she nor her doctor knew there were certain things she was doing that made her risk of developing Alzheimer's greater. I wish she had known. I wish her doctor had known. I wish I had known.

> The first question I asked Katy after the new microwave was installed was, "How's the new microwave working out?"
> "She doesn't use the microwave anymore. I just warm the coffee for her myself."

LDL Cholesterol

Let me give you an illustration of how LDL cholesterol affects the arteries. A friend asked if he could borrow my Swiss Army pocketknife. He had gotten a splinter in the palm of his hand the day before. We were in the back country of Alaska, and his hand was reddened and swollen. The splinter had imbedded itself in the tissue underneath the skin. He could see it but couldn't get to it. He was going to have to take the point of the knife and make a little cut in the skin in order to get it out. I volunteered to help, but he wanted to do it himself. As he stuck the point into the hole the splinter had made, he said, "My body doesn't want it in there."

He was absolutely right. The palm of his hand had become a battlefield. Once a foreign object gets underneath the skin, the body begins sending fluid filled with soldier-type cells to attack the foreigner. If the splinter is not removed, one of two results of the inflammation process occurs. Either the inflammation becomes so severe that the skin ruptures and the battlefield drains to the outside, or the soldier cells begin forming a thick fiber around the splinter, resulting in thickened scar tissue.

The same thing happens when an LDL cholesterol particle gets into the wall of an artery. That LDL particle is like a splinter, and it causes the body to send an army to the battlefield within the wall of the invaded artery. Just like with a splinter, one of two things happens. Either the area swells with inflammation and ruptures inside the artery, forming a clot, or the battle ensues until cells surround the enemy LDL particle and wall it off, forming a scar. Such scarring is known as plaque. My friend's body didn't want the splinter in his palm, and neither does a body want LDL cholesterol "splinters" in the walls of its arteries. The LDL cholesterol splinters do not pick and choose which arterial wall they are going to invade. The battle goes on throughout your body, but when it happens in the heart or brain enough times, you end up with a heart attack or stroke.

The damage takes years to accumulate but usually recurs numerous times at the same places, especially where there is turbulence in the blood flow where an artery divides or where a smaller artery branches off from a larger one. If there is repeated healing and scarring, plaque buildup results until it finally gets large enough to cause a complete blockage of the artery, or one of the battles has so much inflammation going on, it ruptures and a clot forms.

Physicians understand most of the locations in the body where this buildup happens over and over for years and years.

That is why we can say that 85 percent of everyone over the age of fifty has significant blockage within the arteries of their heart without having any symptoms. It is an ongoing and silent process, and it is also happening in the brain. You want to do everything you can to keep the arteries supplying your brain healthy. To do that, you start by changing your food choices. Saturated fat in the food you eat is one of the primary causes of increased LDL cholesterol in your blood. Saturated fat comes mainly from red meat, cheese, butter, cream, and fried foods. Run from them like your mental performance depends on it, because it does.

A study reported in *Current Alzheimer Research* showed that *there was a "significant positive association" between LDL cholesterol and the amount of beta-amyloid plaque found in the hippocampus as well as in other parts of the brain.* The more LDL cholesterol in the blood, the more beta-amyloid plaques in the brain.

Mrs. Dell's thoughts are dimmed by the beta-amyloid plaques and tangles of Alzheimer's. But what else is associated with what is going on? From a medical standpoint, no one knows exactly what causes the plaques to occur. Is the beta-amyloid the cause of the disease? Or is it the result? If beta-amyloid is the end result, then the focus has to be on the cause. Researchers are trying medicines that would possibly prevent the formation of the plaques and tangles or dissolve the plaques that have already formed. But so far nothing has worked. We read in the medical literature that the findings in the majority of dementia patients show a mixture of the beta-amyloid plaques plus disease of the arteries in the brain. In this medical fact, we see a hope that has not been stressed before.

That hope consists of the fact that there are things that can be done to prevent the vascular part of the problem. There are lifestyles that we have control of that can defeat those arterial risk factors.

Mrs. Dell's thoughts are dimmed not only because of the plaques and tangles but also because of diseased, damaged arteries. Dimmed by microscopic strokes, so small that the injury shows no signs or symptoms when they happen to her. And unless some type of prevention is done, the light will get dimmer and dimmer.

Mrs. Dell's Alzheimer's was progressing year by year. It was getting more difficult to interact with her in a normal way. The people she seemed to remember the most were those she had spent time with in past years. I hoped she would always be able to recognize and communicate in some way with the ones who loved her the most—her children and grandchildren.

Her grandchildren came to see her. Each time one was introduced to her by name, her response was the same: "I know, I know."

I knew she was faking it. The grandkids didn't. And that was probably good. It was an excellent weekend. We went to her favorite restaurant and talked and laughed. Each grandchild got to reminisce about the memories they had of her. She smiled and nodded and said she remembered each one.

After lunch, we went back to the patio. The grandchildren continued telling her about good times they remembered. Then I realized she wasn't telling any stories. Oh, she would start a sentence or two and then stop. It was like she could see the words hanging in front of her, but she couldn't grasp them and link them to her tongue. I had seen it many times before. Her thoughts were slow to form, and by the time they got to her mouth, they had been sabotaged.

I put her difficulty out of my mind and began to think how good it was for her grandkids to be there, how good it would be for them to look back at the pictures they were taking, to remember talking with their grandmother and how beautiful she was, to remember what she was wearing, how her hair was done in a special way, and her smile, to remember her while she could still talk *as if* she remembered every word they said.

HDL Cholesterol

Doctors rarely talk to patients about the importance of a higher level of HDL cholesterol for the health of their arteries. Doctors usually talk about LDL cholesterol. There are many fewer HDL particles in the total cholesterol number than LDL, so when the doctor speaks of total cholesterol, HDL gets overlooked. What I want you to remember is that HDL is as important as LDL in understanding how damage to our arteries comes about and what can be done to protect them.

Cholesterol is a double-edged sword. I think if there were some pill that could raise HDL, it would be prescribed as often as the LDL-lowering pill. I say this because the American Heart Association places a significantly low HDL in the category of being a primary cause of heart disease.

A low HDL, below a designated point, is as bad as hypertension or obesity when it comes to potentially having a heart attack. The number 40 is the cutoff, but this is mentioned just to emphasize that the lower the number of the hero HDL cholesterol, the fewer particles to carry off excess LDL cholesterol you have. You want as many extra HDL particles as possible to attack the LDL cholesterol. Doctors should stress that exercise and losing weight raise HDL because there is no medication doctors can write a prescription for. By heeding the advice in this book, you'll know how to improve your hero HDL cholesterol to protect the arteries going to your brain and in the brain itself.

HDL and Memory

HDL cholesterol can actually reduce the amount of LDL in your blood. But does it play a role in our mental abilities? If my HDL were high rather than low, would I score better on those mental tests given to people being followed for MCI or Alzheimer's?

We find part of the answer in a study of over 3,500 men and women in which their HDL cholesterol levels were measured.

The participants were followed for five years, and at the end of the study, *the individuals who had the lowest HDL levels scored the lowest on the memory tests while the higher HDL participants scored higher.* There could be several explanations for these results. Higher HDL could have a protective effect on the arteries in the brain, lessening chances of stroke and arterial damage because of its effect on the LDL particles. Or high HDL could possibly have a direct effect on preventing the accumulation of beta-amyloid. Or it may even have an anti-inflammatory or antioxidant effect on the brain's neurons. But whatever the process, the individuals who had the higher HDL cholesterol scored higher on their mental testing than the ones with lower amounts.

There is so much we don't know about what causes the beta-amyloid plaques or what direct effect each causative factor plays in the development of Alzheimer's. Neither is there absolute understanding how certain risk factors play a role in the disease.

However, we can look at different lifestyles within different groups of people and compare one against the other. It can be shown that a group that exercises performs better on their mental testing than a group that doesn't exercise. Similarly, two groups of people can be evaluated according to their diet. It can be shown those who eat properly do better on their mental testing than the group who eats improperly. And even more definitive, following these groups of individuals eight or ten years down the road reveals that the groups who have the improper lifestyles end up with a higher percentage developing Alzheimer's than the groups who practice the proper lifestyles.

These studies inform us. They show us that most people who develop Alzheimer's have certain risk factors within their lifestyle. Likewise, what happens if these risk factors are avoided? Eliminated?

There is so much information about Alzheimer's that points us in the right direction, that is informative enough that we can get on the proper road until the proof is established.

How HDL Cholesterol Works

If your HDL level is below 40, you are placed into the medical category of cardiac danger. Here is the way to picture what is going on within you.

Think of HDL particles as a patrol car that cruises through your blood searching for lethal LDL cholesterol splinters. The HDL patrol car pulls up by an arterial wall that has several LDL splinters in it and arrests them, puts them into the back of the patrol car, and takes them to jail—the liver—which disposes of them.

Then the HDL goes back to pick up more LDL splinters to carry to the liver. The more of these patrol cars you have, the better. As a matter of fact, for every one point you increase your HDL cholesterol number, you decrease your chances of having a heart attack by 2 to 3 percent. That's why HDL is extremely important.

We have no medications that can increase your HDL. And even if there were, wouldn't you prefer to change your lifestyle rather than taking some pill that might have side effects? We will get specific concerning how certain lifestyles increase your HDL, but for now, imprint on your mind that the two main things you can do to increase your HDL are exercising and losing weight. Additionally, in this book you will learn a third way to improve your HDL. But for now, focus on exercise and getting to an ideal weight as being essential in increasing your HDL level.

There is an excellent article in the medical journal *Circulation* that speaks directly about the HDL "patrol car" mechanism of clearing the lethal LDL cholesterol from the arteries and carrying it to the liver "jail" to be disposed of. The article points out that "the concentration of HDL cholesterol is inversely associated with the risk of developing cardiovascular disease." Researchers explained that it happens by the HDL transporting LDL to the liver to dispose of it. They conclude that "HDL directly protects against the development of atherosclerosis." This study centered on disease of the heart, but other research shows that the same process that affects the health of the arteries to the heart also affects the health of the arteries in the brain. Again the reminder: *what is good for the heart is good for the brain.*

There was a different tone in Katy's voice. "Mrs. Dell doesn't know what clothes to put on, which ones to wear to work in the garden or if we are going shopping. I guess it's a good thing she can get dressed, right? At least she can still dress herself."

Katy walked over to where Mrs. Dell was sitting in her chair
by the large window in the living room and began brushing
her hair and singing to her. As I watched, Mrs. Dell started
smiling, and I knew she didn't have a care in the world.

The Importance of the Ratio of Total Cholesterol to HDL Cholesterol

The cholesterol number that is often the least explained
is the ratio of total cholesterol to HDL cholesterol. If you
were to divide your total cholesterol number by your HDL
cholesterol number, the more HDL cholesterol you have,
the lower that ratio would be. This shows the importance
of having as much HDL as possible to fight the battle and
as few LDL enemies to fight against.

Let's say that in your total cholesterol number there is one
unit of HDL and four units of LDL. If you add them together,
you would have five units for your total cholesterol. If you
divide your total cholesterol by your HDL, you would get a
ratio of 5.0. Now let's say you have two units of HDL and four
units of LDL, giving a total of six units. If you divide your
total cholesterol of six by your HDL of two, your ratio falls
to 3.0. You want your ratio to be below 3.5. Even if your LDL
stays the same, you can drop your ratio by raising your HDL.

The importance of the ratio of total cholesterol to HDL
makes you realize the significance of HDL cholesterol.
Cholesterol-lowering medications affect only the LDL cholesterol part of the picture. If you avoid foods that contribute

to your LDL number and at the same time lose weight and exercise, which increase your HDL number, you will improve your ratio. There is so much more you can do to protect your arteries than take a pill to help lower your LDL cholesterol. Don't focus on one aspect of the battle. Fight the full fight. Look at the whole picture of what is happening and go after quality health.

No medication can protect you as much as you can protect yourself by taking proper care of your body. Statins have been shown to prevent many heart attacks by lowering a person's LDL cholesterol. If your doctor has you on such a medication, by all means take it, but be sure to talk to your physician about your commitment to make lifestyle changes that should make it possible for you to decrease or even eliminate the medicine. Your physician will keep a record of your total cholesterol to HDL ratio. Aim high and shoot for a ratio below 3.5.

Medical research shows that *an increase in your lethal LDL cholesterol and a decrease in your hero HDL cholesterol will take years off your life* because of the effect they have on the disease process in the arteries of the heart and brain. Heart attacks and strokes are the result. Both can be a quick death. But what about Alzheimer's? What about beta-amyloid formation? The first evidence of a direct relationship between LDL and HDL cholesterol in the blood and the deposition of beta-amyloid in the brain was reported in the *Journal of the American Medical Association Neurology.* Researchers found that higher levels of LDL and lower levels of HDL were both associated with greater brain beta-amyloid. In their concluding remarks, researchers pointed out that *LDL and HDL cholesterol levels "had the same pattern of association with beta-amyloid levels as they do with coronary artery disease."* In other words, levels of LDL and HDL cholesterol are as significant in the beta-amyloid buildup causing Alzheimer's as they are in the plaque buildup in the arteries of the heart that causes heart attacks. The problem with Alzheimer's is the slow, slow progression of the disease.

An excellent article in the medical journal *Circulation* pointed out that "the concentration of HDL cholesterol is inversely associated with the risk of developing cardiovascular disease." Researchers concluded that "HDL directly protects against the development of atherosclerosis," which as you recall is a thickening of the walls of the arteries that decreases the blood flow through the arteries. This study centered on disease of the heart, but other research showed that the *same process that affects the health of the arteries in the heart also affects the health of the arteries in the brain.* What is good for the heart is good for the brain.

"When I saw you coming, there was something I wanted to tell you, but I forgot what it was." As she greeted me, Mrs. Dell's pleasant smile was the same as always. "Give me a minute. I'll think of it. Oh, now I remember . . . You remember Sheila who lived next door? She and her two little girls came by yesterday. I told them you were coming today. She said to tell you hello for her."

Mrs. Dell walked ahead of Mr. Dell and me as we continued toward the house. Mr. Dell whispered to me as we followed her, "We know them well. She couldn't remember the children's names." He paused before whispering even softer, "I'm afraid her battery is running down, if you know what I mean."

Cholesterol and Arterial Blockages

The lethal LDL cholesterol splinters floating around in the blood do not pick and choose which arterial walls to invade. Battlefields form throughout the body, but they usually form where there is a turbulence in the blood, such as where a vessel divides or where a smaller artery branches off from a larger one.

The largest artery in the body is the aorta, which travels from the heart, through the chest, and down through the abdomen before evenly dividing, sending blood into both legs. At such divisions, the flow of blood becomes a little turbulent. It is in areas like this that the LDL cholesterol gets into the wall of the artery and begins to cause inflammation and plaque buildup. When this happens at the division of the aorta, there is less blood flow into the legs because of the blockage, and the leg muscles don't get enough oxygen to function properly.

Patients have been referred to me who have developed "window shopper's disease." Medically, it is called intermittent claudication. A patient who has a blockage in one of the arteries to a leg will begin having cramps in the calf muscle of that leg because it is not getting enough oxygen when they are walking. The patient will tell me they have to stop every twenty or so steps to allow the calf muscle to rest. After a brief rest, they can walk another twenty paces before having to stop again. They may use the excuse with a shopping companion that they are stopping to look in a store window. The calf muscle tells a person there is a blockage in the artery by causing pain to get their attention. The muscle can't function anymore unless you stop to let it rest and catch up on its needed oxygen. "Window shopper's disease" is simply a heart attack of the calf muscle in your leg. The only difference is, pain in the leg isn't going to kill you. It lets you know the muscle needs more oxygen and nutrients to continue functioning at the required pace, so you pause to allow the calf to rest until there is sufficient blood flow to get it working again.

When the same type of blockage occurs in the arteries supplying the heart, a person has chest pain called angina. If they stop what they are doing and rest, the heart muscle may react similarly to the leg muscle at rest. After it gets enough oxygen and nutrients, the pain subsides. However, the blockage from the plaque remains and will eventually worsen. The person can have bypass surgery or a stent placed through the blockage in the artery to increase the flow of blood.

Similar blockages are probably forming within the arteries of the brain. The problem is, the person may not know this damage is happening. There is no angina warning pain in the brain. There is no window shopper's warning pain in the brain. Worse, even if the person knew an artery was partially blocked, arteries in the brain cannot be bypassed, nor are we able to place stents in the blocked arteries.

Blockages in the brain's blood supply occur in two areas. One area is the two large arteries that supply the brain, the carotid arteries in the neck. The second area of blockage is the small arteries within the brain itself. Let's look at the large arteries first.

About halfway up the side of the neck the carotid artery divides in two, half of it going to the brain and the other half going to the face. The carotid artery looks like the letter Y when it divides, and this is the most likely place the lethal LDL cholesterol splinters get into the wall of the artery, forming a plaque that decreases the amount of blood that reaches the brain cells. I have operated on numerous carotid arteries and removed the plaque. I have held the plaque in the palm of my hand. The plaque that hasn't been there long can feel soft like butter. But sometimes the plaque has been present so long that calcium deposits have collected, resulting in a hardening of the plaque.

Blockage in the small arteries in the brain is called cerebro-vascular disease. Such blockage is also caused by LDL choles-terol and also decreases blood flow to the cells of the brain. When this happens, there is a much smaller area of the brain blocked from receiving the needed oxygen, and that can result in a mini-stroke that causes only transient problems with such things as speech, swallowing, or the thought process. If the blockage is small enough, you may not even know a mini-stroke happened. Only scarring forms from the injury. In such a case, if a brain is studied, there may be multiple white scar areas even though the person has not had any symptoms of having a stroke. As discussed earlier, this blockage can result in silent strokes or a massive stroke.

Disease of both the large arteries and the small arteries deprives the brain of the blood it needs to function at peak performance. Medical research shows how important it is to keep both the large and the small arteries healthy to prevent Alzheimer's.

If I could do only one physical examination to assess the health of a patient's arteries, I would check the pulse on the top of their foot. The small artery on the top of the foot is the most distant artery from the heart. If it is pounding with a strong beat, that means the arteries between the heart and the foot do not have significant blockage. It also means that the rest of the arteries in the body are most likely open and allowing good blood flow. But if that artery, called the dorsalis-pedis artery, is not pulsating, there is blockage upstream that is preventing the artery from filling. Many times that means other arteries throughout the body have plaque buildup in their walls. If there is not good blood flow to the feet, most likely there is not good blood flow to other parts of the body, including the brain.

A University of Edinburgh study tested older people and found that *those who showed blockage in the arteries going to the legs had lower scores on Alzheimer's mental reasoning tests. They were also 57 percent more likely to develop Alzheimer's within the next eight years.*

This study is a reminder that the LDL cholesterol splinters affect all the arteries throughout the body. If there is blockage in the arteries of the heart, there is likely blockage in the brain. If there is blockage in the arteries of the legs, there is likely blockage in the brain.

I live in the country and have a well with a pump that delivers water to my house. I want the pump as strong as possible and the pipes as clean as a whistle. Both are important in keeping the water flowing properly. A report in the *Journal of Clinical and Experimental Neuropsychology* pointed out what happens in the development of Alzheimer's when both the pump and the pipes—the heart and the arteries—are not working together optimally.

This study included individuals who had no signs of Alzheimer's symptoms but did have disease in the arteries of the heart as well as disease in the arteries from the heart to the brain. None had experienced a previous stroke. The participants' problems included the following:

75 percent were on a statin drug to treat high cholesterol

88 percent were on blood pressure medication

73 percent had known blockages in the arteries of the heart

42.9 percent had suffered a heart attack

32.8 percent had undergone a bypass operation

22 percent had diabetes

14 percent had at least one stent in a heart artery

All of these items are risk factors for healthy arteries. Looking at the people who were on statins or blood pressure medicine makes you want to take notice if you are presently taking a cholesterol-lowering medication or blood pressure medicine.

The individuals in this study underwent mental testing as well as MRI brain studies to evaluate the progression of the disease.

The study looked at two items in the arterial system. The first area of interest was the health of the heart's arteries. Researchers measured the amount of blood the heart pumped with each beat and the total amount it pumped in a given period of time. Of course, the better the arteries of the heart, the more efficient the heart.

The second area of study was the health of the arteries carrying blood to the brain. These were the arteries between the heart and the brain. Researchers assessed the health of these arteries by measuring the thickness of the carotid artery walls. The more LDL cholesterol plaque present, the thicker the wall. This thickness affects blood pressure, which also could be evaluated. Researchers took detailed measurements to determine the amount of blood flowing to the brain.

The third component of the study centered on the MRI pictures of the brain itself. Researchers wanted to see if MRI findings correlated with whether an individual had disease in the arteries of the heart as well as the arteries leading to the brain.

The study concluded that *both the arteries of the heart and the arteries leading from the heart to the brain were associated with mental testing decline and the structural changes of Alzheimer's as seen on brain MRIs.* Their findings also showed that both the impaired pumping output of the heart and the diseased arteries resulted in less blood flow to the brain. Both the pump and the pipes affected the flow.

The takeaway was that a diseased heart and partially obstructed arteries both cause changes in the brains of individuals who don't yet have the symptoms of Alzheimer's.

If you are on a cholesterol-lowering or blood pressure medicine or have had a stent placed in a heart artery or have experienced a heart attack, please make a commitment to do something to change your risk factors and increase the flow of blood to your brain. Your cholesterol matters. Your arteries matter. Your lifestyle habits matter.

One more excellent example from the medical literature to encourage you is found in the medical journal *Neurology*. This article reported findings of a study of individuals who experienced no symptoms of Alzheimer's but did have disease of their arteries. Points were given for each of the arterial problems, and participants were evaluated with MRI brain studies to determine whether they were developing the brain findings of Alzheimer's. Some of the medical problems included evidence of silent strokes, heart disease, carotid artery thickening due to plaque formation, bypass surgery, and lack of exercise.

The individuals were followed for six years. The findings were astonishing. Only 4 percent of the people with the fewest points—the ones with the least amount of disease in their arteries—developed dementia, while 56 percent of the individuals with the highest scores, showing arterial disease, developed dementia. Basically, what this study showed is that *the aging process of dementia is dependent on the health of the arteries.*

Commit to eat properly, exercise, and keep an ideal weight to protect the health of your arteries. To have a healthy brain when you are seventy, you need to eat right and exercise when you are fifty.

"I'm afraid she's getting worse." Katy's eyes did not waver as she spoke to me. "When she and I talk, I don't think she understands me much anymore. I tell her something, and she doesn't respond. Or she gives an answer that makes no sense at all." Katy never wanted to make things sound too bad about the one she cared for like a mother. She continued, "I just want you to know I love Mrs. Dell. I listen to her. And even when she is searching for words, I give her my full attention. I just want you to know that."

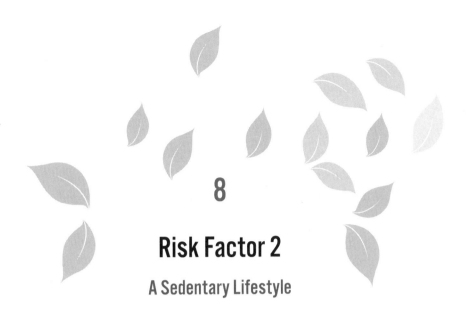

8

Risk Factor 2

A Sedentary Lifestyle

After studying the medical literature, I realized that exercise may be even more significant than diet in decreasing the odds of Alzheimer's. An article in *Lancet Neurology* reported on a collection of studies on the significance of exercise or the lack thereof. The authors of the study concluded that *being physically inactive contributed to the largest proportion of Alzheimer's disease in the United States*. They based their conclusion on evidence that exercise played an important role because of how closely associated it was with other risk factors for dementia. Individuals who didn't exercise were more likely to be obese, have diabetes, and have high blood pressure—all of which result in a greater risk of dementia.

As you can see, the risk factors are intertwined. If you begin a personal exercise program, you will be astonished at how many aspects of your health improve. Exercise is a prime component in losing weight as well as preventing or improving diabetes and high blood pressure.

The report concluded that exercise and the associated risk factors were "all inter-related and probably contribute to Alzheimer's disease largely through vascular mechanism." An article in the *Journal of the American Medical Association* compared individuals who were physically inactive with those who exercised. The study went on for fifteen years, and the conclusion was that *being inactive increased a person's chance of developing Alzheimer's by 50 percent.*

In the journal *Neurology*, a study compared people who were not active with those who exercised at least two times a week. Twice a week is not a lot of exercise, but the results were still amazing. *The people who were sedentary were 60 percent more likely to develop Alzheimer's than the ones who exercised.*

Another study on exercise published in the journal *Neurology* utilized a device worn on the arms of the participants that gave a continuous measurement of their exercise activity. Those with lower overall physical activity had two negative results. One was a higher risk of Alzheimer's, and the second was a faster rate of cognitive decline. The study concluded that *"low physical activity is deleterious to the brain."* (I looked up the word *deleterious*, and here's what I found: harmful, poisonous, deadly, lethal, damaging, destructive, and injurious.) Results like this should motivate you to get moving. You can even watch a football game on television while you are on a treadmill or elliptical machine.

Time and again research shows the importance of exercise in lowering your chances of Alzheimer's. From a medical standpoint, it is important to set up an exercise routine if you don't already have one.

Let's review one last interesting article on the danger of physical inactivity. It is from *Mayo Clinic Proceedings*. Researchers compared individuals who were sedentary, the couch potatoes, with those who did aerobic exercise to sustain their heart rate 60 percent of the maximum rate for their age. Researchers studied the size of the hippocampus, which is paramount to memory, in these people. *The people who didn't exercise had the smallest hippocampus.* Recall that as the nerve cells die, that part of the brain gets smaller. It's no surprise that the people who didn't exercise also did worse on the mental tests that are utilized to detect and follow Alzheimer's.

The report also compared individuals who weren't couch potatoes but whose exercise consisted of simple stretching and toning with those who did aerobic exercise in which they developed a sweat. After one year, the people who did the stretching and toning had less volume in different brain areas than the ones who did the aerobic exercise. Researchers also found that those in the inactive group had more beta-amyloid deposits when studied with PET scans.

How does exercise help lower the risk of Alzheimer's? Exercise is so important in decreasing the chances of Alzheimer's because those who are physically inactive significantly increase their chances of developing the medical problems that increase the risk of damage to the arteries.

From a medical standpoint, inactivity sets up pathways that lead to high blood pressure, high cholesterol, diabetes, and obesity—all of which have a detrimental effect and increase the possibility of Alzheimer's.

Some reports attribute the lower risk to the positive effect exercise has on protecting arteries by elevating HDL cholesterol as well as increasing the strength and efficiency of the heart muscle. Both play an important role in increasing blood flow to the brain. But there are also reports that say physical activity does something even more. Some researchers have found that exercise raises the level of a specific nerve growth factor protein, which is key to brain health, in an area of the brain that is important to memory and learning.

No matter how exercise helps in the avoidance of the symptoms of Alzheimer's, studies show that individuals who do little physical activity have a greater risk of developing this horrible disease. Exercise is something we all should be doing, regardless of whether we know exactly how it helps.

Are you convinced yet? I hope so.

Sitting on the couch and watching television is not the answer if you are trying to avoid one of the most dreaded diseases in the world. If you are a couch potato, your initial program may be walking to the mailbox once a day. Whatever you do, get started. Today is the first day of the rest of your life.

I noticed her gait was just a little different. I hadn't visited her in several months, but I could tell a difference. Did she know what would come next? A walker? A wheelchair? Help getting in and out of her lounge chair? Feeding herself would become difficult, and someone would have to lift the spoon or fork for her. I knew these inevitable events were coming. But she didn't realize that her gait was the initial sign of the coming battle. Alzheimer's is not an easy foe.

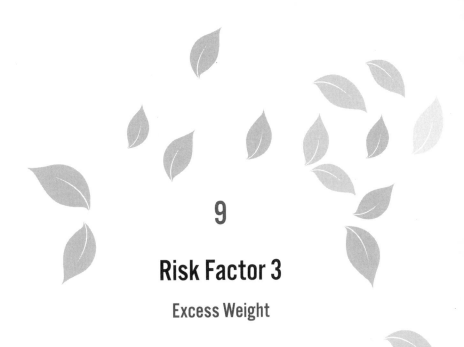

9

Risk Factor 3

Excess Weight

The next time you look at the number on the scale, please take a moment to consider whether it increases your chances of developing Alzheimer's.

In a study published in the *British Medical Journal*, researchers studied 10,276 members of the Kaiser Permanente medical care program of Northern California who volunteered for periodic health checks beginning in midlife. The study covered twenty-seven years and evaluated participants' risks for developing dementia.

The researchers made interesting discoveries about the relationship between excess weight and Alzheimer's. *They concluded that midlife obesity was associated with an increase in the development of stage 2 MCI as well as stage 3 late-life Alzheimer's.*

Let's break down the numbers from a medical standpoint. The report showed that being overweight at age forty to forty-five increased one's risk of developing dementia by 35 percent. Being obese increased the risk of developing dementia by 74 percent. These people were all compared with individuals of normal weight.

Here is the part of the report I found interesting. Having operated on arterial disease for years, I knew that one of the reasons for the increase in the risk of dementia was most likely the effect being overweight has on the arteries. However, researchers suggested an additional problem that fat tissue may cause. Fat tissue may cause an inflammatory reaction within the brain tissue. Their reasoning came about because there is an increase of what is called C-reactive protein in obese people. This protein increases when there is inflammation going on in the body.

I don't want to go too deeply into specifics because so much is unknown concerning the exact cause of Alzheimer's. What you do need to realize, however, is that extra fatty tissue does matter in the beta-amyloid picture of Alzheimer's. These studies accentuate midlife as an important time to commit to improving your health. But in truth, no matter what period of life you are in, it's important to reach your ideal weight.

A report in *Vascular Health and Risk Management* showed a *twofold increase in the chances of a person developing Alzheimer's in late life if they were obese in midlife*. Researchers also studied obesity in correlation with findings on image studies of the brain. An increase in the amount of fat tissue in the body was found to correlate with three factors that are found in patients with Alzheimer's. First, there was a reduced volume in several areas of the brain. Second, there was an increase in beta-amyloid deposits in the brain. And third, there was a decline in mental testing. Being overweight or obese is also one of the main factors in the development of high blood pressure and diabetes, the next two risk factors for Alzheimer's we will discuss. The triad of being overweight, having high blood pressure, and having diabetes all have an effect on the health of your brain.

An article in *Archives of Neurology* reported on a study in Finland that looked at three important risk factors (high cholesterol, high blood pressure, and obesity) and determined how much risk each was in the development of Alzheimer's. The findings showed that the *people who had all three of these risk factors increased their chances of developing Alzheimer's six times more than compared to someone without these factors.* When they broke them down to individual risks, they found that they had an additive effect, with each of them increasing the risk of Alzheimer's by approximately two times.

As we talked, I realized Mrs. Dell could remember things from years ago but not from recent days past. Not yesterday or the yesterday before that. She shared in great detail about the times she sang solo with her choir group. Those memories made her so proud. She remembered their first new car—it was red with gray seat covers. She even told me about the first time she ever ate cotton candy. Pink was her favorite color. She stood in line for the cotton candy at the county fairgrounds, just beside the stand where they threw balls at the stacked bowling pins.

"Now, when did you all get here?" she asked after describing the fair.

"Yesterday," I said hesitantly. "Yesterday afternoon. You were sitting out on the patio when I drove up."

As I drove home the following day, I couldn't help but wonder if Mrs. Dell would remember me being there to visit with her.

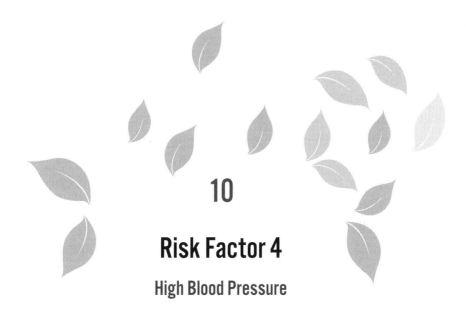

10

Risk Factor 4

High Blood Pressure

A little elevated blood pressure, a little excess weight, too many ice cream bars. Whatever had caused the beta-amyloid to accumulate in Mrs. Dell's brain was continuing its destructive process. It was becoming more and more evident every time I saw her. I began to prepare myself for the report Katy would relate to me each time I visited.

Katy skipped the usual "How are you getting along these days?" as she met me at my car. "There's something you should know." I wondered if she told Mr. Dell all these things or just waited until the next time I was in town.

"What is it, Katy?" She was holding Mrs. Dell's pill box.

"She's not taking some of her medicine. At least every three days she doesn't take the morning pill. I asked her about it, but she tried to convince me she is taking her pills like always.

I don't want to check every pill she is supposed to take, but I don't think she remembers to take all her medicine."

Before I left, I had a good discussion with both Katy and Mrs. Dell. I explained the importance of taking the medicine at the appointed time. Mrs. Dell said she couldn't tell the difference anyway, so she didn't think the medicine was that important. Both finally agreed that Mrs. Dell was still in charge of taking her medicine, but Katy would check the pill box to make sure it was being taken properly. I explained to Mrs. Dell that it was not unusual to forget medicine from time to time but that she should go along with the check-and-balance plan. She agreed.

Six months later, Katy told me that Mrs. Dell was not taking any of her medicine on her own. "She doesn't even remember where we keep the pill box. She asked where the box was for a while, and I would tell her, but now she doesn't even ask. I just give her the medicine as it has been prescribed. And I give every pill she is supposed to get. Every day."

People who are overweight or obese often have two other risk factors: high blood pressure and diabetes. We talk about these three together because they are so interrelated. You may say that you are obese but haven't been diagnosed with diabetes or high blood pressure. Let me just say that if you are obese, either or both of these factors could be on their way without you being aware of it.

The first number in a blood pressure reading is called the systolic number. Imagine your heart squeezing and pumping a large amount of blood into your arteries. They begin to bulge and expand under the pressure. The amount of pressure pushing on the walls of the arteries is called the systolic pressure.

When the heart muscle finishes its contraction and goes into a resting stage, it is being refilled with blood. When this happens, the amount of blood in your arteries is reduced, causing a reduction in pressure against the arterial walls. This relaxed pressure is called the diastolic number.

Normally, these two numbers should read 120 over 80: 120/80. A person is not classified as having hypertension, high blood pressure, until their pressure reads 140/90 or above. But the problem lies in between these two readings. Many people are neither normal nor labeled as having high blood pressure. They are borderline. Their blood pressure is somewhere above 120/80 yet below 140/90. There are degrees of pre-hypertension. A person may be obese and not have high blood pressure, but if they are obese, they are probably on the road toward hypertension.

The same is true with diabetes. Being overweight makes a person much more prone to developing diabetes. Their blood sugar may not be at the magic number that labels them diabetic, but it is above normal. Many obese patients are pre-diabetic.

Your weight is an indicator of so much more than just heaviness. The great majority of obese people are sedentary.

You may not be labeled obese, but if you are overweight, you may as well look at yourself as being "pre-obese" and start following the guidelines we set for weight loss. If you work on losing weight, you are working on the prevention of Alzheimer's. You will be reducing your risk of scoring lower on those mental tests.

Two-thirds of Americans are overweight or obese. These two-thirds need to pay extra attention to the guidelines on weight loss, but even if you are at a normal BMI, you can still be overweight by as much as twenty pounds. For those of you who are at your ideal weight, the studies on obesity will motivate you to maintain this weight.

A study presented in the *International Journal of Obesity* showed the interworking of obesity and high blood pressure. This report covered an eighteen-year period and examined individuals who had no signs of Alzheimer's or other cognitive mental problems at the beginning. None had dementia, a history of stroke, or any heart or arterial problems. Researchers began mental testing four years later and then followed their performance.

The group was divided into two smaller groups. The people in one group had neither an increase in weight nor high blood pressure. Those in the other group were overweight and had hypertension.

As they were followed, those who were both obese and had high blood pressure performed worse on mental tests than those who were neither obese nor hypertensive. The study showed that obesity by itself played a negative role, and high blood pressure by itself played a similar negative role. Those with the best results were neither obese nor had high blood pressure.

The study showed a linear relationship between weight and blood pressure. As a person increased in weight, they had a greater potential to develop high blood pressure and a greater potential to develop the problems that lead to Alzheimer's dementia.

Even if a person is not overweight, high blood pressure is dangerous in relation to Alzheimer's. In fact, one of the highest reported risk factors for dementia is high blood pressure in midlife. In later years, blood pressure may fall because of aging factors, so the best time to correlate the relationship between high blood pressure and Alzheimer's is in midlife. Whatever your age, it is time to cut out the salt.

Observational studies of people who have some type of dementia, including Alzheimer's, have shown that there is an association between midlife high blood pressure and late-life dementia. In fact, up to 30 percent of people who had late-life dementia had high blood pressure in midlife.

High blood pressure can wreak havoc on the brain's mental capacity. It is associated with disease of the large arteries that lead to the brain as well as the small vessels within the brain. An increase in blood pressure can lead to a stroke. As already discussed, some people have silent strokes without even knowing it. Some estimates state that one-fourth of people over the age of seventy have had a silent stroke. These small areas can be seen on MRI studies, and many times there are multiple silent stroke areas. In these areas, neurons die, eventually affecting memory and normal brain function.

A study in the medical journal *Cell Metabolism* made some black-and-white statements concerning high blood pressure and dementia. One statement said, *"Hypertension has devastating effects on the brain, being the major cause of stroke and a leading cause of dementia."*

"Why does Mrs. Dell spend so much time watering her flower garden?" That's what Katy asked me when I walked into the house for a visit. Katy told me that if she didn't walk outside and tell her to come eat lunch, Mrs. Dell simply wouldn't eat. "And right after her meal, she is back out in the yard, holding the hose, giving each plant a hundred times more water than it could ever use."

I wondered if spending so much time in her flower garden was an escape from the mental pressure of Alzheimer's. There was no one to talk to. No one to judge her actions. She didn't have to pause in an attempt to remember the next word in a sentence. There was no stress. In her garden, everything was different. It was relaxed—like Alzheimer's didn't exist. Mrs. Dell was so happy in that garden. She smiled the whole time.

I explained this to Katy. We decided it was best to let her enjoy the garden. "It's like little pieces of her are disappearing, but let her enjoy the bits that are left."

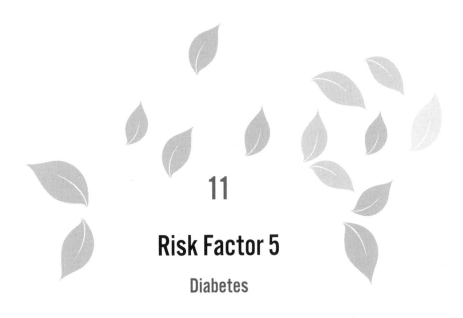

11

Risk Factor 5

Diabetes

The following two statements ought to be a red alert to anyone who is diabetic. They are from a multitude of articles referring to the correlation between diabetes and Alzheimer's.

> Diabetes doubles a person's chances of developing Alzheimer's dementia.
>
> Diabetes accelerates progression from MCI to stage 3 Alzheimer's dementia by three years.

With type 2 diabetes, resistance builds up to the insulin produced in the pancreas. Initially, the pancreas produces excess insulin, but eventually it can't keep up with the need to control the glucose in the blood. This excess insulin leads to an inflammatory response in the cells in the brain. Inflammation is one of the contributing causes of Alzheimer's.

Even more significant is the negative effect diabetes has on the arteries. Diabetes is listed as one of the vascular risk factors that results in decreased blood flow to the nerve components of the brain.

As diabetes develops, a person's blood sugar level goes from normal to slightly elevated. That person is placed into a category called pre-diabetes. When the blood sugar level gets higher, the diagnosis of diabetes is made. When pre-diabetics are studied, we see how diabetes is linked to three lifestyle habits over which we have control: a poor diet, a sedentary lifestyle, and obesity. Studies have shown that pre-diabetic individuals can prevent full-blown diabetes by eating the proper diet, exercising, and losing weight. These are also the three lifestyle choices for defeating dementia.

Smoking

I am adding smoking as an additional risk factor. The reason is because it is in a class by itself as far as causing injury to your body. I can't think of any process that harms the body more than smoking. It is one of the biggest risks there is for your arteries, not to mention the cancer risk. Most everyone realizes that smoking is one of the worst things you can do to your body. We will not go into the details of smoking as related to Alzheimer's except to acknowledge that people who smoke have a greater risk of Alzheimer's. I have cut out lung cancer from many patients and have found there are two types of people who smoke. When told they have cancer of their lung, there are those who will completely commit and quit smoking, and there are those who will continue smoking no matter what their doctor or spouse tells them. I expect the same response from many who smoke when they are informed that smoking increases your chances of developing Alzheimer's.

So, my advice to anyone who smokes is to quit—plain and simple. I have given the same advice to smokers I have operated on. If the lung tumor was not malignant, I informed them that if they didn't quit their pack-a-day habit, they were going to develop lung cancer. It is beyond my reasoning why someone who is headed to cancer of their lung won't quit smoking, but I realize it is up to them to make the decision to change their lifestyle. The same pertains to Alzheimer's. You are soon going to learn the ten-minute factor that will teach you how to break addictions. Whether giving up cigarettes or eliminating the food you shouldn't be eating, you can learn steps to abstain from the bad habits that increase your chances of Alzheimer's.

Mr. Dell hadn't noticed that Mrs. Dell wasn't keeping up with her medicine. He wanted me to explain what was happening.

"It's called stage 3." As we sat on the patio, I began explaining what was going on inside her mind. "She can no longer take care of her daily activities. It really started when her car keys were taken away, but I didn't want to paint such a dark picture of what was ahead. But now that she can't take her medicine on her own, she is definitely in stage 3."

He looked at me with almost a blank stare. "Stage 3? That's the last one, isn't it?"

"Yes, it is."

"Will she get like her mother did? Before she passed?"

"I don't know how bad it will get." I hesitated because I didn't really want to continue. But I did. "No one knows. Alzheimer's is one of the biggest medical mysteries there is. We don't know how long or how far it will go. We will just have to keep encouraging her and wait to see." It was hard to talk to Mr. Dell like this. The future was basically waiting for her to get worse. The day would come when he would come home and there would be nothing left. More and more of her leaves were falling.

He removed his glasses, and his eyes welled up with tears. He lightly wiped the tip of his finger across each corner. He knew what was to come. He just didn't know until now that it was called stage 3.

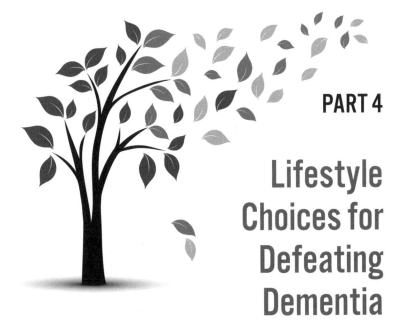

PART 4

Lifestyle Choices for Defeating Dementia

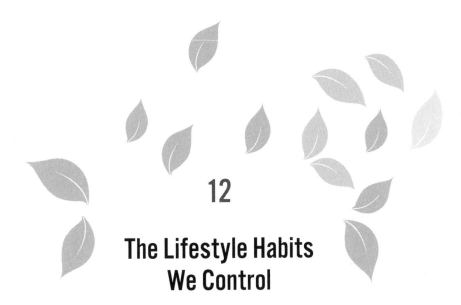

12

The Lifestyle Habits
We Control

The Chicago Health and Aging Project offered some interesting estimates concerning the prevalence of Alzheimer's disease. The study showed that *one in eight people, 13 percent, age sixty-five and older has Alzheimer's, and approximately 45 percent of everyone eighty-five and older has Alzheimer's.*

Just two days after I read the report detailing the above statistics, I attended a conference. I was seated at a table with other attendees, and we were all eating breakfast. The gentleman beside me was pleasant and very talkative. He would be considered at least overweight and possibly obese. We were having a nice conversation when I began noticing what he was eating. His pancake was as large as his plate. But it wasn't just the pancake that caught my attention. He had unwrapped four large pats of butter and laid them evenly around the circumference of his feast. His pancake looked like a clock face with butter at twelve, three, six, and nine. I had never seen that much butter on a pancake in my entire life. Just off to the side were two large pieces of bacon and two links of sausage. I have to admit that I had to concentrate on what he was saying because I was thinking about all those studies I'd been reading about Alzheimer's. That's when I realized there were eight people sitting around the table. Not everyone was sixty-five, but the day would eventually come when all of us would be at least that age. I couldn't help but think about the odds of one of us developing Alzheimer's.

As we talked, I learned that the gentleman beside me was a chef. I didn't say anything to him about the effect the foods he was eating had on the brain, but I realized he didn't know. He hadn't thought about it. He had no idea. He was like Mrs. Dell earlier in life. Perhaps if he knew, he would eat differently.

That's one of the reasons I wrote this book. I want everyone to have the knowledge they need to make informed lifestyle decisions. I believe if you know the factors that place you at a greater risk of developing Alzheimer's, you will work toward developing the healthy lifestyle habits that will lower those risks.

My passion is that everyone will learn how to decrease their odds of developing Alzheimer's.

I believe the information in this section will help you think differently about eating harmful foods. You will begin visualizing exactly what a particular food is going to do to you. I guarantee that you will have less and less desire for bad foods the more you remind yourself what they do once inside your body.

After learning what the medical literature says about excess weight and exercise, you will have a yearning to get to your ideal weight. You will want to exercise rather than sit on the couch. You will look at life from a different viewpoint. I changed my lifestyle habits when I realized how my choices would affect my body in the years to come. Medical knowledge changed my life forever, and I am hopeful it will do the same for you. I believe that the more you know about what is going on in your body, the easier it will be for you to change how you live. I promise it will be easier to avoid the risk factors that lead to Alzheimer's now that you understand the connection between those risk factors and Alzheimer's.

The following statement spells hope: *most risk factors involved in the onset and progression of Alzheimer's are modifiable.* Apart from genetic risk factors for Alzheimer's, the factors we've covered are all related to the health of your arteries, and when you change your habits, you can decrease your likelihood of Alzheimer's. Three lifestyle habits can help you deal with every modifiable risk factor for Alzheimer's.

Your success in the battle against Alzheimer's comes down to whether you exercise or not, what foods you eat and don't eat, and whether you are overweight. You can't separate one risk factor from the others, and you can't pursue one crucial lifestyle choice in isolation from the others. They are all interrelated. They are intertwined. Each one helps the others. The good part is that when you commit to the best hope for preventing dementia, succeeding in one lifestyle habit leads to success in the other two.

Being overweight has some relationship with not exercising and how you eat. Being diabetic or having high blood pressure is often related to obesity. Not exercising can be related to them all. So our warfare against Alzheimer's is not a one-on-one match. It requires taking all you've learned about the risk factors and understanding which of them you may be dealing with. It also involves modifying your lifestyle into a healthy way of living. We are going to cover each lifestyle choice, and you will learn how the habits work together to fight the controllable risk factors for Alzheimer's.

You Can't Control Your Genes But...

So many people attribute everything to their genes. But even if you inherit some bad genes, you can still decrease your odds of developing Alzheimer's.

Watching Mrs. Dell over the years made me wonder if I should be tested to see if I had any genes that would increase my chances of developing Alzheimer's. I knew the APOe4 gene, which is fairly common, doesn't cause Alzheimer's but can increase the likelihood of developing it.

I asked myself what I would do differently if I found out I had the APOe4 gene. Would I get a PET scan to see if I had beta-amyloid plaques forming in my brain? Would I get an MRI to see if any part of my brain was getting smaller?

Would I have my spinal fluid tested? And if I did have the gene, and if my PET scan was positive for beta-amyloid plaques, and the MRI showed less volume, and my spinal fluid showed a lot of tau protein and very little beta-amyloid, would I do anything differently?

Knowing there is no medication that can cure Alzheimer's, I definitely would begin doing everything possible to fight the problem. I would work hard to develop a lifestyle that protected the blood flow to my brain.

I would immediately change my eating habits. I would avoid the foods that increase the LDL cholesterol splinters that cause disease of the arteries in my brain. And in place of the bad fats, I would not substitute sugar but would concentrate on eating the good fats instead of the bad. I would make eating fish a habit.

I would exercise to increase my HDL cholesterol. And I would zero in on my ideal weight and retain it forever.

That's what I would do if I were tested and found to have a gene for Alzheimer's.

It became clear to me that I should do the same things whether I have a bad gene or not. The same positive lifestyle habits are good for my heart, my brain, and my entire body. I should do all I can to maintain a healthy body. It's the only one I have.

I did not want to go through what Mrs. Dell was experiencing. Watching Mrs. Dell progress through the disabling process was the best textbook I ever read on the prevention of Alzheimer's.

I was told Phyllis had come by to see Mrs. Dell the day before I arrived. She was one of Mrs. Dell's closest friends. Phyllis was about twenty years younger than Mrs. Dell, but they did many fun things together. Phyllis played the piano at the church where Mrs. Dell sang in the choir. They had frequently traveled together and made so many good memories.

"Do you remember when I was in college and offered to cut your grass?" I asked Mrs. Dell. Her smile was instantaneous.

"I do. We had just bought our first riding lawn mower. I hadn't even ridden on it once."

"Mr. Dell wasn't home, but you showed it to me and I got it started without a hitch. Do you remember what happened?"

"The tree stump."

"Yes, the one you didn't tell me about."

"Don't try to blame that on me," she was quick to respond.

"I bent the blade so badly that the mower stopped."

"Brand-new," she said. "I remember it well."

It was fun sharing many laughs together. Today Mrs. Dell was having a great day. I hoped we could experience many more days like today.

"I understand Phyllis came by to see you yesterday," I said.

"No. She didn't come by." There was no longer a smile on Mrs. Dell's face, only frankness—like I had said the wrong thing. "No, Phyllis hasn't been by to see me for quite a while actually. I was just wondering the other day why I hadn't seen her."

I realized I had been too hopeful. I needed to accept the fact that some of her neurons were dying every day.

Developing the Proper Habits to Minimize Risk Factors

Someone told me the other day that 43 percent of a person's daily lifestyle depends on the habits they have developed. I say "developed" because we have control over the routines we do every day. Repeated practice leads to habit formation. Your eating habits are just that: habits. You either have a habit of eating between meals or you simply find it awkward. You have a habit of either exercising or not each day that comes around. If you do not have a habit of exercising five to six days a week, you will have to make the decision every day, and the odds that you will exercise are markedly against you.

The problems associated with high cholesterol, a sedentary lifestyle, excess weight, high blood pressure, and diabetes are all related to how you handle your lifestyle habits. Whether you eat properly, maintain your ideal weight, or exercise is dependent on the habits you develop. So much in life is related to habits. Your routines eventually become habits that you don't even think about. Willpower and self-discipline are the two most important factors in the success of habit development. You have to remain focused and disciplined for success in developing proper lifestyles.

A Healthy Diet

Decision time happens before you eat. Go over your eating plans again and again until they become ingrained in your mind. Know what you are going to do when the moment comes when you think about eating a snack. The same is true with mealtimes. Before you put food on your plate, know the amount you are going to eat and don't go back for seconds. Decide before the meal that there will be no dessert.

To combat Alzheimer's, you have to develop the proper eating habits. Period. You don't want to have to make a decision every time you sit down to eat. Eat a certain breakfast out of habit. Develop two or three healthy lunch options, and eat them out of habit. Once you develop your proper eating habits, you won't have to think about what you're eating. When you learn the right eating habits while you are losing weight, you won't have to change anything when you reach your ideal weight. You will maintain that weight the rest of your life—out of habit.

Create habits around healthy choices. Decide to always eat fish instead of steak. Always pass on the cheese, butter, and high-fat salad dressing. Always choose grilled over fried. Soon your wants will change, and you will be in the habit of eating a healthy diet. Your eating culture changes. To lose weight, develop the habit of centering your eating on fiber, fruits, and vegetables.

Pick an alternative for every bad food you want to eat. Substitute fish for steak. Instead of a hamburger, eat a salad with grilled chicken. Substitute high-fiber cereal or oatmeal for bacon and eggs. You need to eat three meals a day, but just substitute the good for the bad.

Make your meals habits rather than a series of choices. Breakfast is the easiest. Lunch is almost as easy. Don't look at a menu to choose something new, look at a menu to find what you are in the habit of eating. Don't look at a menu for ten minutes. Look at it for one minute and look, out of habit, for one of three items you are planning to eat.

When you want a snack, abstain for ten minutes, drink some non-caloric beverage, and get busy doing something else. At first, you may feel an urge to eat, but you control how you react to it in your mind.

Ideal Weight

Willpower and self-discipline play a major role in weight loss. Don't fall for diet schemes or advice from friends who lost weight through a special way of eating. Most weight-loss diets do actually help people lose weight, but the problem is that over 88 percent of the time a person regains a significant portion of the weight.

Realize that fruits, vegetables, and fiber make you feel full with the least amount of calories. Develop the habit of eating these foods as your major source of energy. Develop healthy eating habits while you are losing your excess weight, and when you get to your ideal weight, your habits will follow you the rest of your life. Your habits will help you sustain your ideal weight.

Exercise

Exercise is the one lifestyle habit that influences the other habits the most. When you exercise, you begin to feel better, you begin to lose weight, and you begin to eat differently because you don't want to undo the good you have just done. You begin thinking differently about weight loss and what you are doing to your arteries and about getting seven to twelve years younger physiologically. You get better at regulating your "want to" in your life. Exercise strengthens your goals to the point of success.

If you write down what you are going to do, your goals are much more likely to happen. Write down when and where you are going to exercise each day and what that exercise will consist of. What clothes you will wear. Which running shoes. Think about the obstacles you may face and develop a plan of action. Write out your plan of action for the reward you will receive with each accomplishment. Write it out and look forward to your reward once you have succeeded in reaching your goal of what to eat and of finishing your exercise for the day.

When we look at the factors that can increase the risk of Alzheimer's, we realize there is hope. All of the risk factors can be affected by the lifestyle habits we control. Exercising, eating properly, and sustaining a proper weight are important in protecting the arteries, both of the heart and the brain.

Ronald Petersen, director of the Mayo Clinic Alzheimer's Disease Research Center and the Mayo Clinic Study of Aging, sums it up best: "We've been preaching for years that what's good for the heart is good for the brain." He goes on to say, "Maybe our efforts to watch our diet and exercise are having a spillover effect, leading to less dementia."

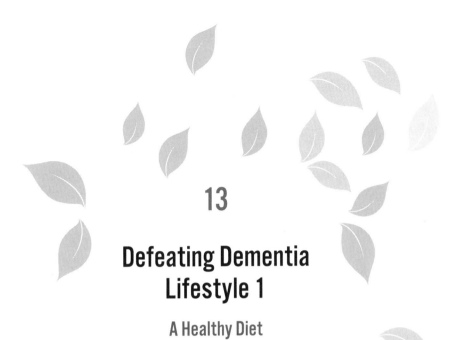

13

Defeating Dementia Lifestyle 1

A Healthy Diet

A special report published by the editors of *Focus on Healthy Aging* made a statement that is being confirmed in more and more brain studies. The fact that a healthy diet leads to a healthy heart is uncontested. Increasingly, researchers are proving that many lifestyle factors that help protect the heart help protect the brain as well. The report stated, *"Some of the same conditions that make a person more susceptible to heart disease also make dementia more likely."* This is another way of saying, "What is bad for the heart is bad for the brain."

One of the factors that affects both the heart and the brain is diet. What we eat and don't eat has a huge impact on the health of the arteries in the brain. The diet that has been studied the most in relation to a reduced incidence of Alzheimer's disease is the Mediterranean diet. It emphasizes a high intake of fruits, vegetables, legumes, peas, nuts, fish, and olive oil. It also emphasizes a low intake of red meat, dairy products such as cheese, butter, and cream, and foods fried in animal oils.

An article in the Alzheimer's Association's publication studied MRI results of people who ate the Mediterranean diet compared with those who didn't. The study looked at individuals who had no symptoms of Alzheimer's whose mean age was 79.8 years. The MRI study measured the thickness of four areas of the brain to determine if those who ate the Mediterranean diet had thicker brain mass in those areas compared with those who ate red meat, cheese, cream, and butter and who did not eat fish, nuts, and olive oil.

The MRI study revealed that *a higher adherence to the Mediterranean diet was associated with a larger, thicker cortical portion of the brain.* They attributed the findings to healthy arteries as a result of the Mediterranean diet.

Research showed just the opposite with high red meat intake. A higher intake of saturated fat in red meat correlated with more disease in the arteries of the brain. Other studies showed that *high red meat intake was detrimental in dementia.* The MRI study mentioned above substantiated this finding by observing an association between red meat and less thickness of the cortex area of the brain.

Another Mediterranean diet study reported in the medical journal *Neurology* looked at 674 elderly individuals who did not have symptoms of dementia. They were followed with MRI studies of the brain to measure the deteriorating shrinkage of the brain as a result of beta-amyloid accumulation. One group ate the Mediterranean diet, and the other group did not. The study found that *those who adhered to the Mediterranean diet had less brain shrinkage.* This study showed that two elements contributed to the benefits of the diet on the structure of the brain: higher fish intake and lower red meat intake. It is as important to eat fish as it is not to eat red meat.

The journals *Neurology, Archives of Neurology, American Journal of Clinical Nutrition,* and *Annals of Neurology* published articles that addressed how the foods we eat and those we avoid play a role in the development of Alzheimer's. They all showed the advantage of eating the Mediterranean diet.

One of the studies reported that people who ate the Mediterranean diet had a 28 percent lower risk of developing stage 2 Alzheimer's and a *48 percent lower risk of progressing from stage 2 to stage 3.* Recall that stage 2 begins with the initial symptoms and persists until the person has to depend on someone else in order to carry on normal activities. Stage 3 begins when independence is lost and extends for the remainder of the person's life. If Mrs. Dell had eaten the Mediterranean diet in her earlier years, she would have had a 28 percent lower risk of developing stage 2 Alzheimer's. And even if she had symptoms, the diet would have lowered her risk of progressing to stage 3 by 48 percent. The concluding statement read, *"Higher adherence to the Mediterranean diet is associated with a trend for reduced risk of developing MCI and with reduced risk of MCI conversion to Alzheimer's Disease."*

In the journal *Frontiers in Nutrition*, another study reported "that higher adherence to a Mediterranean type diet is associated with slower rates of cognitive decline, reduced conversion to Alzheimer's disease, and improvements in cognitive function." That is a great statement for anyone in stage 2 Alzheimer's who has begun having symptoms but has not yet lost their independence. Even if they have begun to decline in reasoning and memory function, their diet can improve cognitive function or at least slow down decline.

"Mrs. Dell, you are beautiful. Your hair makes you look like a queen today." I stood by her chair, smiling at her.

She lifted her head only slightly, but her eyes looked directly at mine. She raised her eyebrows, and the biggest smile showed on her face. She said nothing, but her smile said it all. I knew my trip to see her was not in vain—she recognized me.

The Prescription for Life Diet

My Prescription for Life diet is similar to the Mediterranean diet, but the Prescription for Life diet is a little more strict for a very good reason. While the Mediterranean diet emphasizes *moderation* in regard to red meat, cheese, and cream, the Prescription for Life diet emphasizes *abstaining* from these foods. The reason is simple: food is an addiction, and if you don't overcome the desire, you will eventually return to your former ways of eating.

Let's use smoking as an example. Everyone realizes that smoking is an addiction. There is no way to quit without defeating the desire for a cigarette. You can't tell yourself that you are going to smoke only one day a week. Switching to a cigarette that has a reduced amount of nicotine will not take away your desire for the one you usually smoke with high nicotine content. You can't beat an addiction unless you defeat the desire for that substance. Abstinence is the only way to defeat an addiction.

I grew up eating red meat. Steak, hamburger, and pork ribs were all a part of our evening routine. But today if you put a steak on one plate and salmon or grilled chicken on another, I do not have even the remotest desire for the steak. The more I abstained from eating red meat, the easier it became to avoid it. After about two months of abstinence, the desire begins to leave. Six months later, you are un-interested in that food.

You are not going to beat your desire to have steak by eating leaner cuts or grass-fed beef, just as you are not going to eliminate your desire to smoke by smoking light cigarettes. You will not overcome the desire for cheese by eating low-fat cheese. It won't be long before you stop telling your server to leave the cheese off your sandwich or your salad. Your desire for cheese will return just as it used to be—unless you abstain.

The Prescription for Life diet differs from the Mediterranean diet in the following ways because of the addictive factor:

1. No red meat rather than a small amount.
2. No saturated fat rather than a small amount.
3. No cheese, cream, or butter rather than a small amount.

The Prescription for Life diet emphasizes fruits and vegetables, whole-grain cereals, peas, beans, nuts, pasta, fish, and olive or canola oil. The foods to avoid are red meat, cheese, cream, butter, and fried foods. Each of these is high in saturated fat.

Years ago, I read an article in the medical literature concerning saturated fat that changed my eating habits for life. It stressed that we get most of our saturated fat from cheese. Cheese doesn't necessarily have the highest content of saturated fat, but we eat so much of it that it ends up being the source of the largest amount of saturated fat we consume. At that time, cheese was my favorite food, especially pepper cheese. I was a connoisseur of cheese. All my patients knew how much I loved it. There was a small cheese factory near my town, and every Christmas I would receive numerous gifts of cheese from my patients.

As a surgeon who operated on diseased arteries, I knew the significance of that report. I knew that saturated fat is the source of LDL cholesterol. I knew that LDL cholesterol is the cause of disease in the arteries. I realized that my favorite food, cheese, was contributing to the greatest amount of saturated fat in my diet. I put the article down and never ate cheese again.

If you like the idea of prevention, the one item to avoid at all costs to protect the health of the arteries in your brain is saturated fat.

To stress this point, let's look at a study of women's health that evaluated two groups. One group consisted of women who ate the most saturated fat, while the second group ate the least amount. Both groups were intermittently given mental tests to see how they scored over time. The results revealed that *the women who ate the most saturated fat had the worst scores on their mental tests and were about 65 percent more likely to show a declining score on their mental tests over time.*

Other studies showed even more significant findings concerning how much saturated fat a person eats. These studies showed that participants who ate the most saturated fat not only did poorly on mental tests but also had an increased risk of developing stage 2 MCI as well as stage 3 Alzheimer's dementia. In the medical journal *Archives of Neurology*, a follow-up study of 815 individuals without symptoms of Alzheimer's found that *people who ate the most saturated fat had 2.2 times the risk of Alzheimer's compared with those who ate the lowest amount.*

Mr. Dell passed away a few days ago. Mrs. Dell went to the funeral, but there were no tears, no sign that she understood what was happening. It was just an event she attended.

The Good Fats

While it is important to abstain from the foods that contain saturated fat, it is just as important to eat the foods that contain the good fats: omega-3, polyunsaturated, and monounsaturated. The good fats come in fish, nuts, and olives. Salmon is the best, but any fish or seafood is better than steak. We are talking grilled fish rather than fried. Walnuts and almonds are the best nuts, but any nuts are better than cookies or donuts or candy bars. Olive oil or canola oil should replace butter in all of your cooking.

We know that eating the good fats—omega-3, polyunsaturated, and monounsaturated—plays an important role in the health of the arteries and preventing heart attacks and strokes. But what about Alzheimer's? The more I read about the significance of the good fats in fish, the more I decided I needed to form the habit of eating fish as much as possible.

Research reported in *Archives of Neurology* studied 815 individuals over sixty-five who were initially unaffected by Alzheimer's. The study went on for seven years. Researchers compared the people who developed Alzheimer's with those who didn't and also kept record of how much fish each person ate. The findings were astounding: *the participants who consumed fish once or more per week had a 60 percent less risk of Alzheimer's disease compared with those who rarely or never ate fish.* This was a fact I couldn't ignore. Researchers found this to be a linear association, meaning that the more fish a person eats, the less risk of Alzheimer's. Those within *the group who ate the most fish had a 70 percent reduction in their risk for Alzheimer's.*

Eating fish for the health of the arteries is emphasized by three significant organizations. The Centers for Disease Control and Prevention, the American Heart Association, and the American Stroke Association each recommend eating fish two to three times a week, primarily for arterial health. But now research points out that reducing vascular risk factors may not only reduce disease of the arteries in the brain but also decrease the deposition of beta-amyloid in the brain.

An interesting study in the *Journal of the American Medical Association Neurology* evaluated whether eating fish helps reduce the formation of beta-amyloid deposits in the brain. Researchers performed brain scans to evaluate the volumes of brain areas that are usually affected by Alzheimer's.

I want you to memorize an acronym. The letters are DHA. They stand for an omega-3 fatty acid called docosahexaenoic, one of the good fats found in fish. After reading about this report, you will want to eat a lot of it.

Basically, this study correlated four items for each participant:

1. The amount of DHA each individual had in their blood sample as a result of eating fish

2. A PET scan of the brain to see how much beta-amyloid was present

3. An MRI study of the brain to evaluate the amount of viable brain cells present in certain areas to see if there were areas with less brain mass due to the death of cells

4. Mental tests to evaluate Alzheimer's progression

Here's what the study found. *The individuals with lower levels of DHA in their blood had a greater deposition of beta-amyloid in their brains. Those with higher DHA levels in their blood had larger brain volumes in the areas of the brain that are typically involved in Alzheimer's, such as the hippocampus. Those with higher DHA levels in their blood also had higher test scores.*

Another interesting study conducted at Tufts showed similar results concerning fish. Almost nine hundred older men and women who did not have any symptoms of Alzheimer's were given mental tests every two years to see if any of them developed symptoms. Anyone who developed symptoms was classified as having stage 2 MCI or stage 3 Alzheimer's dementia. They were followed for nine years to see what effect eating fish had on their mental acuity.

This study focused on how many servings of fish were consumed per week. *Those with the highest levels of DHA ate an average of three servings of fish per week.* Those who ate less fish had lower DHA levels in their blood. The people who ate the most fish, resulting in the highest levels of DHA, had a 47 percent less risk of developing stage 2

MCI and a 39 percent less likelihood of developing stage 3 Alzheimer's.

One of the most referred-to studies concerning fish and DHA is the Framingham Heart Study. As reported in the journal *Neurology, the higher the level of omega-3 fatty acid in the blood, the lower the risk of dementia.* Researchers measured the amount of DHA in the blood of the participants. They also did brain-imaging studies and mental testing. What they found was that the individuals who had beta-amyloid deposits had 23 percent less DHA in their blood than the ones who did not have beta-amyloid deposits. Those who had higher DHA levels had a greater brain volume in certain areas of the brain that are related to memory. And last, the people with higher DHA levels did better on the mental tests.

Just one more quick example of how the good omega-3 fat in fish affects the brain. Researchers conducted MRI studies on the hippocampus, correlating its size with the amount of fish individuals ate. Mental tests were also performed. Two groups were studied: those who ate the most fish versus those who didn't eat fish.

The people who ate fish on a weekly basis had greater volumes of nerve cells not only in the hippocampus but also in the frontal and temporal lobes, which also are related to memory. As far as the mental testing went, only 3.2 percent of those who ate the most fish went on to develop the symptoms seen in MCI or Alzheimer's dementia, while 30.8 percent of those who didn't eat fish developed cognitive decline regarding their test scores. The concluding statement stressed the importance of eating fish to increase the brain's resistance to Alzheimer's disease and lower the risk of dementia.

At one time, I thought that if I ever took a supplement, it would be omega-3 because so much in the medical literature pointed to the benefit of this good fat found in fish. An article in the journal *Clinical Interventions in Aging* impressed upon me the importance of eating the fish. The article reported on several clinical trials that investigated the effects of omega-3 supplements on Alzheimer's: all failed to demonstrate that supplements help prevent Alzheimer's disease. So let's agree to eat the fish, and many reports encourage us to eat at least three servings a week.

One evening I pulled up a stool next to Mrs. Dell's chair. We chatted about what life was like growing up. She seemed to remember about earlier days.

Then out of the blue she looked at me and said, "Albert will be home in just a little while."

I didn't know what to say. "You remember Mr. Dell has passed away, don't you?" I took her hand in mine and gently rubbed it. I continued, "He was such a great man. So kind and generous. Everyone loved him. I know how much you loved him." She just looked at me.

A slight smile began to form on her thin lips. "Yes, I know. You are right. He was such a good man. I really miss him."

Sugar

When you avoid certain foods, you will naturally substitute other foods in their place. Studies show that if you substitute processed sugar for the bad fat, you are not helping your arteries. The number of heart attacks and strokes doesn't change all that much. Eating more donuts and cake rather than red meat doesn't change the equation as much as substituting salmon for steak.

Quite a bit of media coverage stresses the evils of sugar rather than of fat. They say sugar causes the problems with the arteries rather than fat. They are half right, but remember that a half truth is a whole lie. It is not just the sugar but the bad fat *plus* the extra sugar that causes damage to the arteries.

One study compared people over seventy who ate the most carbohydrates with those who ate the least amount. Those who ate the most carbohydrates had nearly four times the risk of developing MCI than those who ate the least amount.

An article in the *European Journal of Clinical Nutrition* showed the consequences of substituting sugar rather than monounsaturated and polyunsaturated fats for the bad fat. *Those who replaced saturated fat with monounsaturated and polyunsaturated fats rather than carbohydrates significantly affected their cognitive decline, equivalent to delaying aging by about four to six years.*

Make this your rule: bad fat is an enemy and sugar is an enemy. Do not substitute refined sugar for the bad fat you quit eating.

Fruits and Vegetables

One article pointed out that elderly people with the highest levels of vitamin B1, B2, B3, B12, C, D, and E in their blood scored higher on mental tests than those who had low levels. The best way to get these vitamins is to make sure your diet is high in fruits and vegetables. Don't depend on supplements; eat the whole food that contains all the fiber and other nutrition that goes along with the vitamin load.

There was an interesting article from Rush University about vegetables. Researchers studied cognitive decline in relation to the amount of vegetables individuals ate per day. According to the results on the mental exams, two servings of vegetables a day was the equivalent of the prevention of five years of mental aging. Over a period of six years, researchers compared people who ate less than one serving of vegetables a day to individuals who ate 2.8 or more vegetable servings a day. *Those who ate the most slowed their rate of cognitive decline by 40 percent.*

I want to take you back to medical school to learn a little physiology of how brain cells communicate with each other. This will explain one reason why eating fruits and vegetables may help in fighting Alzheimer's.

As you recall, the little fingerlings extending out of each neuron allow the neurons to communicate. The tips don't actually touch, but there is some material that "connects" the two extensions, allowing one neuron to send messages to another. This communication connection is called a synapse. The blood-brain barriers are the thin protective walls between the bloodstream and the brain cells. These barriers are important in allowing certain factors to pass through from the blood to the brain cells as well as allowing other factors to flow back out of the brain. Vegetables and fruits, especially berries, have a substance that can cross the blood-brain barriers, and it is believed to benefit the synapses, allowing communication between brain cells. It does so by cutting down on inflammation and acting as an antioxidant to prevent oxidation at these areas of communication between the brain cells. Think of oxidation and inflammation as rust around the ends of the cells. Fruits and vegetables are the best antioxidants and anti-inflammatories you can ever feed your brain.

Alcohol

There is a lot of discussion about alcohol and health. This discussion usually centers on the relationship between drinking in moderation and the health of the heart and the arteries. Most studies recommend no more alcohol than two drinks a day for men and one drink a day for women. Studies on alcohol and Alzheimer's show that alcoholism, the drinking of too much alcohol, is one of the risk factors contributing to Alzheimer's. But how much is too much?

Studies show that heavy alcohol consumption has a deadening effect on neurons that leads to brain damage. Many chronic alcoholics show significant damage in their brains. A Finland study reported on 554 twins whom researchers followed for twenty-five years. They found that binge drinking at least monthly in midlife was associated with more than a threefold increase in the risk of dementia after the age of sixty-five.

A statement published in the medical journal *Circulation* gives good advice: "Unlike other potentially beneficial dietary components, the consumption of alcohol cannot be recommended solely for vascular risk reduction. Alcohol can be addictive, and high intake can be associated with serious adverse health and social consequences, including hypertension, liver damage, physical abuse, vehicular and work accidents, and increased risk of breast cancer."

The bottom line: if you don't currently drink alcohol, don't start.

Meal Platforms

I hope the studies we examined convinced you of the importance of a healthy diet in decreasing the risk of Alzheimer's. Now let's look at the specifics of a healthy diet.

Breakfast

Fiber is what breakfast is all about. The main lesson to learn concerning fiber is that the kernel, the outer covering of a grain, is what provides the most fiber. In foods commonly defined as whole grain, the kernel is left intact and therefore more fiber is present. Fiber One cereal has the highest fiber content of the common cereals. Most cereals have 2 to 4 grams of fiber, whereas Fiber One has 14 to 16 grams, depending on which type you choose. A good alternative for a high-fiber breakfast is steel-cut oatmeal. In steel-cut oats, the outer covering is intact and provides extra fiber. Even on those mornings when you decide not to eat cereal, you can get some fiber by eating whole-grain toast with jelly. Of course, if you are toasting the bread yourself, don't add butter. If you are ordering toast at a restaurant, be sure to specify dry toast or it will inevitably be drenched in butter.

In medical journal articles about foods you should eat, fruit is consistently mentioned. Breakfast is the easiest time to get in over half of your fruits when you are aiming for a combination of five fruits and vegetables a day. Add strawberries, bananas, blueberries, or raspberries to your cereal, or simply put fruit in a bowl and eat it along with your whole grain toast.

On the breakfast platform, you will use skim milk with zero saturated fat. Almond milk, soy milk, and rice milk contain no saturated fat, so your LDL cholesterol will not become elevated.

Next on the breakfast menu is egg whites. There are two reasons not to eat the egg yolk. One is the amount of saturated fat in it, and the other is the amount of dietary cholesterol in it. Egg yolk has the most concentrated amount of dietary cholesterol of any food we commonly eat. The American Heart Association recommends that if you have diabetes, high cholesterol, or heart disease, you should limit your daily cholesterol intake to no more than 200 milligrams a day. Since you are developing an eating lifestyle of prevention, be proactive and limit your dietary cholesterol before you develop diabetes, high blood cholesterol, or heart disease. When you order an egg-white omelet, specify no cheese or the odds are it will come to your table with cheese included.

Lunch

Time and again, the medical literature highlights two food groups as healthy choices: fruits and vegetables.

Why do fruits and vegetables always make the list? Why are they always discussed in connection with losing weight? First, fruits and vegetables make you feel full with the fewest calories. But even more important is the fact that fruits and vegetables are nearly void of the bad fat that causes an elevation in LDL cholesterol. It is easy to incorporate fruits and vegetables into your diet by eating a salad for lunch. A salad that includes peas, beans, and nuts is a good choice.

For a sandwich, use grilled fish or chicken. If you order a sandwich at a fast-food restaurant, ask for no mayonnaise or cheese. Anytime you can get some type of fish for lunch, as long as it is not fried, order it. Eating fish three to five times a week is a good goal.

Instead of French fries, order a baked potato. Leave off the butter and sour cream. Add pepper to the potato and then mash it with your fork. (Or you may find other interesting ways to eat a baked potato that you will like.)

A bowl of vegetable soup emphasizes the "goods" rather than the "bads." Any non-cream-based soup is a good side item.

What do you drink with your meal? One rule of thumb, whether you are in the weight-loss portion or the weight-sustaining portion of your plan, is this: no calories from liquids. Develop a habit of drinking water or tea or any other drink that has zero calories. The calories in liquids are hidden calories you never think about.

Dinner

For most people, dinner is the main meal of the day. It usually begins with a salad followed by the main course and then possibly a dessert or a cup of tea or coffee. Your new lifestyle will certainly differ from that of most others, but beginning with a salad is still a good start. Whether at home or in a restaurant, there are many salad combinations to choose from. Be sure to choose a nonfat dressing to avoid hidden saturated fat.

Grilled fish is still the emphasis. I can't stress enough how important it is to eat the healthy fat found in fish. Fish is the double-barreled shotgun in fighting disease of the arteries. It lowers the unhealthy LDL and raises the healthy HDL.

When you order grilled fish at a restaurant, remember to ask your server to place the sauce on the side so you can determine whether it is cream or cheese based, which you will want to leave off. Salmon is the best choice and is found in most restaurants and grocery stores. Other fish such as tuna and trout also contain the good fat, as do lobster and shrimp.

For something different, whole-grain pasta is a good alternative. There are habits you need to develop when ordering anything Italian. Rather than cheese or meat sauces, ask for simple tomato-based marinara. With whole-grain pasta, you are not only avoiding saturated fat but also eating the high fiber you need for your intestines.

Let me mention one treat my wife and I enjoy occasionally. We order it at a small restaurant that specializes in pizza, and they know what we want when we walk in. Our server just smiles and nods her head. The pizza she brings has no cheese, just the usual marinara that comes on all the pizzas. But on top of the thin, crispy crust are some pieces of spicy chicken, strips of fresh pineapple, and caramelized onions. If you try, you can get very creative with a cheese-less pizza.

Snacks

During the weight-loss portion of your new eating life-style, there should be no snacks at all. Remember, snacks, even good snacks, contain calories. Snacks are extra calories that will add on weight.

Snacks are permissible once you reach your ideal weight and do not have to control your calories as much. The best snacks consist of fruits or nuts. Keep some grapes in the refrigerator, along with some nuts in the pantry. You can change your choices for snacks today. You do not need to remember that walnuts and almonds are a little better than peanuts. Just quit eating cookies, pastries, and ice cream and begin eating any type of fruit and nut. Nuts contain the good monounsaturated fat that raises your HDL cholesterol. They do contain some saturated fat, but the large amount of good fat outweighs the bad.

Food Lists

Good Foods and Good Fats

Vegetables, fruits, salads, legumes (beans, peas), nuts, whole-grain pasta, high-fiber cereal and steel-cut oatmeal, non-cream-based soups, olives, olive oil, canola oil, fish, monounsaturated fat, polyunsaturated fat, omega-3 fat.

Bad Foods and Bad Fats

Red and processed meat, cheese, egg yolk, cream, ice cream, cream sauces, cream-based soups, butter, margarine, fried foods, saturated fat.

Sample Meals

Breakfast
- foods high in fiber (cereal, steel-cut oatmeal, whole-grain toast)
- fruits
- skim milk
- egg whites

Lunch
- salads
- fruits
- vegetables
- grilled fish or chicken
- baked potato
- non-cream-based soups

Dinner
- salad
- grilled fish or chicken
- whole-grain pasta or cheese-less pizza

Snacks

- fruits
- nuts

A Picture for Your Mind

Don't kid yourself when dealing with your most prized possession. There are many ways we hedge on medical truthfulness when it comes to eating. "I will eat only half a slice of that butter-filled cake," we tell ourselves. "Moderation is the rule I am going to live by," we say. "I bought this at the organic food store, so it must be good for me." The rationalization goes on and on.

Keep your eating habits simple. You are learning the difference between the bad fats and the good ones. This platform will help you choose cereal over bacon, eggs, and biscuits with gravy for breakfast; a grilled chicken sandwich with a baked potato over a cheeseburger and fries for lunch; and fish over steak for dinner. Base your eating habits on what food does to the aging process of the body.

I want to paint a picture in your mind of the foods you should avoid that play a significant role in the damage to the arteries going to the brain.

A Big, Juicy Steak

Picture yourself sitting in a nice restaurant as the waiter brings you an oval plate with a big, juicy steak on it. This represents the red meat—beef, pork, and lamb—that you are going to avoid. Saturated fat is highest in these meats. The day will come when you won't even want to buy or order them because you know what such food does to the arteries that supply your brain. Your desires will change.

You hear that center-cut bacon, which is cut next to the bone, has less saturated fat than other bacon. You hear that leaner cuts of beef have less fat than others. You even hear that grass-fed beef is much better for you than all the others. These things may be true to a minute degree, but what you want to imprint on your mind is that certain foods are dangerous to your arteries and other foods are not. You are learning a habit of avoiding certain food types. You want to avoid the types of foods that contain saturated fat, which is known to rob you of your health.

A Fried Egg Sunny-Side Up on Top of the Steak

Your waiter comes by and adds a fried egg sunny-side up on top of the steak. Egg yolk is a high-cholesterol food, with one jumbo egg yolk containing 270 milligrams of dietary cholesterol. Compare that to four ounces of beef containing 100 milligrams, and salmon with only 70 milligrams, and better yet, tuna with only 40 milligrams.

A Slice of Cheese on Top of the Egg

The waiter places a big slice of cheese squarely on top of the steak and the egg. As I told you earlier, at one time cheese was my favorite food. My patients knew how much I liked it and brought me all types of cheese as Christmas gifts.

Then I read a journal article explaining how the saturated fat in cheese causes an increase in LDL cholesterol, which is a primary cause of blockages in the arteries of the heart and the brain. By the time I finished reading the article, I had made the decision to quit eating cheese. I hope you have just made the same decision.

A Glass of Whole Milk to the Right of the Plate

In your mind, picture the steak on the plate, the egg on top of the steak, and the cheese on top of the egg. Now see your waiter place a glass of whole milk beside the plate. If you look closely, you can see little specks of pure cream floating on top of the milk. Milk is rich in nutrients and the calcium your bones need, but whole milk contains a great deal of fat. The good news is that you can easily buy, drink, and cook using skim milk from which the fat has been removed.

Whole milk contains about 4 percent butterfat. That reads as 6 grams of saturated fat on the nutrition facts label. The fat has been removed from skim milk. It doesn't take a genius to figure this one out. If you want to decrease the amount of fat you put into your body, begin using skim milk—or almond milk or soy milk—on a routine basis.

I recall when I first realized how much fat is in whole milk. I read that the fat in a glass of whole milk is equivalent to that in five strips of bacon. I will never forget drinking my first glass of skim milk. It tasted like water. I was sure it was a taste I would never grow to like. But I kept thinking about fatty bacon, and it wasn't too long before skim milk tasted normal and a sip of whole milk made me wonder why I ever liked it in the first place.

If you look at a quart of whole milk that has not been pasteurized, you will see that the cream has risen to the top of the container. Whole milk you buy in the store contains that same amount of pure cream, just mixed in with the rest of the milk. So when you think of milk, also think of that cream in your mind picture.

That takes ice cream out of your eating lifestyle.

As well as cream sauces restaurants want to pour over your grilled fish.

As well as cream-based soups.

As well as so many desserts that taste so good.

A Pat of Butter to the Left of the Plate

The waiter now places a pat of butter on a small plate to the left of the large plate. Butter has two things you want to avoid: cholesterol and saturated fat.

Many people suggest substituting margarine for butter because margarine doesn't contain cholesterol. But margarine still has about the same amount of saturated fat as butter. Butter and margarine both fit into the bad picture. So quit putting either butter or margarine on your bread and your baked potato.

Rather than butter or margarine, use substitutes such as Benecol or Promise Activ. These are cholesterol-lowering spreads. Also use olive oil and canola oil in cooking. They contain the good monounsaturated and polyunsaturated fats. If you want to put something on your bread, put some olive oil on it.

Many of the sauces on the foods you order are butter or cream based. You may order grilled fish for dinner, but with it comes a thick, cream-based sauce that is loaded with butter. You will learn to avoid the creamy Alfredo sauce and ask for a marinara or basil sauce instead. Once you learn who the enemy is, you will think differently about what foods you eat.

Grease Poured over the Food

For the final piece in your mental picture, the waiter brings out a small plate with a polished silver bowl in the center and sets it before you on the table. You look into it and see a blob of grease. He then picks up the bowl and pours the grease on the butter, then into the glass of milk, and then on top of the slice of cheese. Part of it splatters onto the tablecloth, while the rest runs down over the egg and the steak and mixes with the yellow egg yolk floating on the bottom of the plate. He places the little silver bowl back on its plate and walks away. As he leaves, he turns his head and states two words: "Nothing fried."

What a great reminder. The basic oil used today in frying food is animal based and full of the saturated fat you want to avoid. That silver bowl of grease represents many of the foods you now eat. But from this day on, you will put these fried foods on a scale and weigh the outcome of what will happen to the arteries in your heart and brain if you continue consuming them as you do now. Just think of all the fried foods you eat. French fries, fried fish, fried chicken, and the list goes on and on. Down South, they even eat fried green tomatoes. To learn from this portion of the picture, begin thinking grilled rather than fried, not only because of the bad oil used in the frying but also because frying a food adds about a third more calories than grilling. Grilling cuts down on calories as well as saturated fat.

The waiter is gone, and now you have the picture that will help you remember about 90 percent of the foods you are going to eliminate from your diet. You don't have to quit them all at once, but you want to begin working on the entire picture. Doing so protects not only your heart but also your brain.

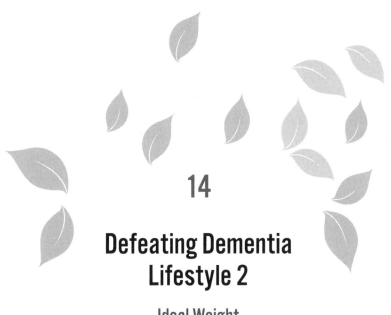

14

Defeating Dementia Lifestyle 2

Ideal Weight

Reaching your ideal weight is so important because being overweight causes so many problems most people simply do not realize. Most individuals connect excess weight with their appearance, but extra body weight is a billboard calling attention to the fact that other problems are likely going on: high cholesterol, high blood pressure, physical inactivity, and diabetes. Many studies in the medical literature also show a direct correlation between body weight and mortality. The rate of mortality increases with the more weight added. If you are not obese but are overweight, don't pat yourself on the back, because the damage progresses one pound at a time.

Body mass index is a measurement utilizing a person's weight and height. A BMI of 20 to 25 is considered normal,

25 to 30 is considered overweight, and over 30 is considered obese. An article published in the medical journal *Obesity* provides scary numbers for anyone who is overweight.

> Obesity in midlife is associated with approximately double the risk of late-life dementia.
>
> Being overweight in midlife is associated with approximately a one-third increased risk of late-life dementia.

A report in the journal *Neurology* provided even worse numbers: "*Obesity in midlife is associated with a 3.08 times increased risk of Alzheimer's for women and a 2.45 times increased risk for men.*"

Medical professionals have long known that being overweight has a negative effect on the arteries to the heart and the brain. We are now learning about the role weight gain plays in contributing to the problems in the brain that lead to Alzheimer's. A profound statement appeared in *Current Alzheimer Research*. Study results were "consistent with prior reports that *midlife obesity at 40–55 years increases the risk of developing clinical dementia and Alzheimer's disease in later life.*"

An article in *Archives of Neurology* reached a similar conclusion. Researchers studied 2,047 adults without dementia and followed them with MRI studies to evaluate their brains. BMI was used to determine obesity. Researchers found that those who were obese in midlife developed Alzheimer's in later life more often than those who were not obese. Another article in *Archives of Neurology* had the same conclusion: *"Obesity at midlife is associated with an increased risk of dementia and Alzheimer's Disease later in life."*

Have I convinced you yet? These studies all compared individuals who were at their ideal weight with those who were overweight. My mother always told me, "Nothing good ever happens after midnight." I would like to say, "Nothing good ever happens from being overweight." I strongly encourage you to get to your ideal weight.

Being obese increases the risk of a person developing Alzheimer's because so many other health risks are directly associated with being overweight. As an individual's weight increases, so do their cholesterol level, their blood pressure, and their blood sugar, resulting in diabetes. All of these risk factors, individually and combined, lead to the development and progression of Alzheimer's.

The three questions to ask yourself are:

1. What should I weigh?
2. How do I lose excess weight?
3. How do I stay at my ideal weight for the rest of my life?

Mrs. Dell was becoming much less active. She spent most of her time in a wheelchair. She was having one of those days when the dementia seemed to be taking a nap. Several of us sat in her living room watching television with her and communicating fairly well. I was seated in a chair next to her recliner.

Suddenly, her facial expression changed. She looked out the window, then toward the door, and then at me. "It's time for me to go home."

I wasn't sure what to say. "Mrs. Dell, you are at home, and your bedroom is just down the hall." I pointed toward her bedroom. She looked so surprised. "That's your bedroom. Let's get you to bed. I know you are sleepy."

Her face seemed to relax only somewhat as she responded, "I'm not sleepy, but I do need to go home."

I patted her hand and began to rub it gently. Then I helped her into her wheelchair and rolled her to her bedroom. The event reminded me of years ago when I put my children to bed.

What Should You Weigh?

There are several ways to determine your ideal weight. Most medical advice goes by BMI, body mass index. As mentioned, 20 to 25 is considered normal, 25 to 30 is considered overweight, and above 30 is considered obese. Those fairly nonspecific numbers are determined by your height and how much you should weigh on average. You can find free BMI calculators online that will automatically determine your BMI. The problem with BMI is that you can be twenty to thirty pounds over your ideal weight and still be considered within the normal range or the overweight range.

There is a formula I like that is more specific than BMI. It shoots pretty lean but may give you a good number to aim for. You may add five to ten pounds to this number depending on your body build and bone density.

For men, use 105 pounds as a baseline for the first five feet of your height, then add five pounds to that baseline for every inch over five feet. For women, use 95 pounds as a baseline for the first five feet, then add four pounds for every inch over five feet. Again, this gives you an approximate ideal weight, but you will have to fine-tune it for your body build.

If you are overweight, it's important you start losing those excess pounds, but even more important is that you lose them in a way that enables you to sustain that weight loss for the rest of your life. Unless you develop the proper eating habits, your chance of keeping the lost weight off is only 2 to 20 percent. If you develop proper eating habits from the beginning, you can continue them forever.

Katy went to great lengths to make sure they celebrated Mrs. Dell's birthday in a big way. She invited all of Mrs. Dell's friends and caregivers. There was a large cake, balloons, matching birthday plates, and many beautifully wrapped gifts. As everyone sat around the table waiting, Katy rolled Mrs. Dell into the dining room in her wheelchair. Katy led the group in singing "Happy Birthday." Then she cut Mrs. Dell the first slice of cake and placed it in front of her.

Katy noticed Mrs. Dell glance at her as if somewhat alarmed. Then she asked, "Is it *my* birthday?"

How Do You Lose Excess Weight?

Write down the weight you want to reach. Make a commitment to reach it. Put it on a sticky note and place it on your mirror or carry it in your purse or wallet. Your ideal weight is achievable. You can reach it!

I hadn't seen her in almost six months. As I stepped into the living room, I saw Mrs. Dell sitting in her brown leather lounge chair. She was cuddling the dog in her left arm and methodically stroking its back with the palm of her right hand. She immediately smiled at me the moment I walked into the room.

I asked her how she was doing, and she replied, "Fine. I'm doing just fine." She smiled again and continued petting the dog. "How was your trip down off the mountain? Did you get into any of that rainstorm? I saw on television there was a storm headed our way."

I responded that we did have some rain, but three hours ago the sun started shining and we enjoyed the trip down.

"Katy told me the forecast is supposed to be good tomorrow."

She sounded so normal. She knew me. She knew about the weather. She could even remember the next day's forecast.

I walked across the living room and stopped in front of her chair. I was speechless.

The whole time she talked she was rubbing the back of a stuffed toy poodle.

Katy told me later that her dog, Peppy, had died several months earlier and she had bought the poodle to give Mrs. Dell peace of mind and needed companionship. "She pets it a lot." Katy smiled. "Like it's real."

Three Secrets

Here are three weight-loss secrets you can use as soon as you read them.

The first and most important secret in your weight-loss diet is no snacks—period. Nothing between meals or after dinner. Controlling snacks is one of the most significant aspects of weight loss. If you don't eliminate between-meal calories, it will take you a lot longer to lose the excess weight. Here's why. Your body's fuel is glucose. Whether you eat carbohydrates, fat, or protein, your body eventually converts it to glucose. If you feel hungry between meals, it is likely your body's blood glucose level has fallen to a lower level. Your body will get the needed glucose one of two ways. It will break down some of your body fat into glucose, or you will furnish the extra calories through food. Think about that just a minute because it's pretty simple physiology. If you don't supply the need with extra snack food, your body is going to supply the need by burning excess fat.

The second secret is to fill up on fruits and vegetables at mealtimes. These two food groups have lots of fiber that fill you up with the fewest calories. To emphasize the importance of eating fruits and vegetables, some studies encourage five servings of fruits and five of vegetables a day. I encourage at least three fruits and two vegetables a day, but the more, the better.

The third secret is smaller portions. If you're eating at home, this is simple—just put less on your plate and never take seconds. Eating out is a little more challenging. You can split a meal with your spouse or friend. If you order a meal, you don't have to eat everything on your plate. Order light meals. A salad with grilled fish or grilled chicken is filling. Don't eat until you are completely full. Stop and talk for the last ten minutes while you sip on your noncaloric drink. The full feeling will come, but it may take ten minutes or so for you to feel satisfied. Or you can order from the appetizer menu if it offers small portions of (non-fried) fish or chicken and then add a vegetable on the side. An appetizer plus a salad or a non-cream-based soup is even better. There are many ways to decrease portions while on the weight-losing part of the plan. You may even come up with some secrets of your own.

You would be surprised how many people stop me and ask if I would go over some specifics on losing weight. Recently, I did so with one person, and when we finished, he said, "Are you actually saying that I have to cut the amount of food on my plate, eat a lot of fruits and vegetables, and on top of that not eat a single bite of anything between meals?"

Because he was overweight, I wanted to say something positive. So instead of answering him with a simple yes, I smiled, placed my hand on his shoulder, and responded, "I must commend you on your hearing acuity."

> "She doesn't know if it's morning or evening. I have to tell her when it's time to go to bed or she would simply sit in front of the television all night long," Katy said. "Plus, she has no idea which meal it is. She just eats whatever she's fed. She always enjoyed watching her favorite shows on television— she liked *Jeopardy*—but now she just looks all around the TV. And remember how she liked to read? I used to put a stack of magazines by her chair, and she would go through them all day long. Then the reading slowed, and she would look at the same page all day. That's when I started giving her *National Geographic* because she liked to look at the pictures."

The Rules on Losing Weight

Here are a few additional rules to follow when you are attempting to lose weight.

1. No bread before meals. Whole-grain breads do not contain saturated fat, but they do contain sugar. Think

of bread as sugar. Sugar equals extra calories. During the weight-loss aspect of your plan, the less bread, the better. Even if you order a grilled chicken sandwich for lunch, you can remove the bun and just eat the chicken, lettuce, and tomato. Make sure you request no mayonnaise on your sandwich.

2. No appetizers before meals. You may order an appetizer for your main course and add vegetables to it.

3. No desserts. These are completely superfluous calories. If you are in the losing-weight mode, no desserts—period.

4. No second helpings of anything. If you finish eating your portion and are still a little hungry, do not get a second helping. Simply wait a few minutes, and you will feel satisfied. In the meantime, drink a little more calorie-free liquid or enjoy conversation at the table.

5. No calories from beverages. Don't add sugar to your coffee or tea. Even if you live in the South, don't drink sweet tea. Sodas, energy drinks, and sports drinks are the biggest sources of added sugar in the average American diet—accounting for more than one-third of the added sugar we consume.

6. No fried foods. You add about one-third more calories when you fry a food. Go grilled rather than fried.

7. No cream-based soups or fat-filled salad dressings. If you choose salad for lunch, ask for fat-free dressing on the side.

Early on, Mrs. Dell used a walker. She could walk to the nearby patio to enjoy her favorite sitting place.

However, the time of using a walker was short, mainly because of her balance. Then she graduated to a wheelchair. She could be pushed out to the patio but needed help getting in and out of the wheelchair. That lasted for several years.

She could transfer from the wheelchair to the car with a little help. Cracker Barrel was her favorite restaurant. I don't know if it was the food or the fact that they had a big, round table just as you entered the dining area that she could easily roll her chair up to without making a fuss.

Then the day came when we couldn't get her into the car. And then came the day when Katy and the other caregivers couldn't move her from her living room chair into the wheelchair. That was the day I realized what bedridden really meant. It was a life-changing day. That was the day I realized that many of her leaves had fallen.

The Ten-Minute Factor

Let me tell you one more secret for losing weight. I learned this from a gentleman in Alaska who in his younger years had three addictions: drugs, alcohol, and cigarettes. He quit them all and shared with me how he did it. He called it the ten-minute factor. I have used it with my patients who needed to lose weight or quit smoking. Here's how it works.

My friend said that anyone can control an addiction for about ten minutes. When he quit smoking and wanted a cigarette, he would tell himself that he wasn't going to smoke for the next ten minutes. Then he would get busy doing something else, like watching TV, working in the yard, calling someone, or reading a book. After a while, the desire for a cigarette would come back, and he would repeat his ten-minute factor.

The key to beating an addiction is to *beat the desire*. Food is an addiction. Try the ten-minute factor and quit eating the wrong foods. Use it to lose excess weight. Make the rule of no food whatsoever between meals or before bedtime. If you crave a snack while attempting to get to your ideal weight, decide not to eat the snack for ten minutes. Pour yourself a glass of noncaloric liquid and do something to take your mind off the snack. After about two months of applying this marvelous secret, your desire for certain foods or your desire to snack before bed will be gone. I promise that once you have beaten the desire, you have beaten the addiction.

How Do You Stay at Your Ideal Weight for the Rest of Your Life?

One morning you will step on the scale and realize you reached your ideal weight. You may even do a victory dance. Your eating habits will not change. That is the key to not regaining the weight you lost. You learned what foods lower your chances of developing Alzheimer's. You changed your desire concerning what you eat. If you decide to eat a snack, you choose fruits or nuts, not the sugary snacks you once desired.

Here is the most important key to maintaining your ideal weight once you have lost the excess: your weight-loss eating habits must remain as weight-maintaining habits.

Your goal is not simply to get to your ideal weight. Your goal is to maintain that ideal weight for the rest of your life. If you don't, the plan has been a failure. A report in the *National Weight Control Registry* stated that only 2 to 20 percent of people who lose weight are able to keep it off. Would you buy a stock that gave you only a 20 percent chance of making a profit? Would you take a medication prescribed by your doctor if they told you it worked only 2 percent of the time?

Quick-fix fad diets are even worse. On such diets, 95 percent of the people who lose weight not only regain it but also add more pounds to it within a three-year period.

One more lifestyle habit will help you reach and maintain your ideal weight: exercise.

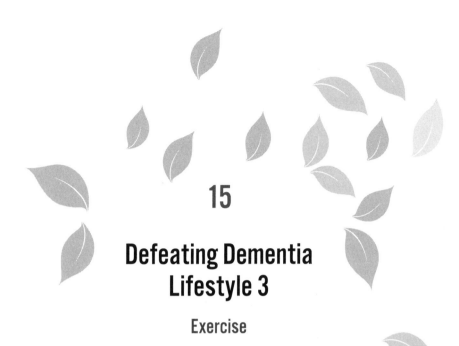

15

Defeating Dementia Lifestyle 3

Exercise

I wish Mrs. Dell had developed an exercise routine back when she was first diagnosed with Alzheimer's. It would have been even better if she had done so when she was forty, or even earlier. But she didn't have any idea the importance exercise would have for her future.

Regular physical activity is more effective in reducing the risk of Alzheimer's than any drug available.

Katy kept Mrs. Dell as mentally active as possible. She played *Jeopardy* games with her, asking questions Mrs. Dell would know the answers to. She showed Mrs. Dell pictures of flowers in *Better Homes and Gardens* and asked her to name them.

She sang one of Mrs. Dell's favorite songs and ten seconds into it asked Mrs. Dell to join in.

During one of my visits, we were sitting around talking, as usual. I kept thinking Mrs. Dell was having one of her good days, but suddenly her mind switched into another mode. Her tone was anxious and bordered on anger. "Where is he? Why wasn't he home to greet you all when you arrived? He should be here." She began looking around as if he were hiding somewhere. "You just wait. Albert will be here soon. He's supposed to be back any minute now."

"Mr. Dell passed away, Mrs. Dell. You remember . . . he's gone."

"You know how pretty my roses have always looked. They are my favorites. I may get some help watering them when he gets home." Her mind changed direction.

I felt I should say something to reassure her. "I know you have forgotten, but Mr. Dell passed away and won't be coming home again. You'll get to see him again in heaven someday."

The skin on her face suddenly became creased. Her eyes squinted like she didn't believe me. Her whole demeanor turned into an expression of astonishment and sorrow before she finally spoke. "What happened to him?"

"He had a heart attack. He didn't suffer." I was afraid she was about to start crying.

She sat stunned. Then her face returned to normal, and she just looked toward me—not at me—like she actually acknowledged something was wrong with her reasoning. Like she should have known her husband was dead. Like she should have remembered.

Exercise and the Brain

A study in the journal *Healthy Aging Research* revealed that exercise resulted in a significant increase in the size of the hippocampus in a group of females. As you know, the hippocampus is a primary part of the brain involved with memory. Researchers compared the individuals who exercised the most with the ones who exercised the least. They concluded, *"Individuals with the lowest 10% of daily activity were reported to have a two-fold higher risk of developing Alzheimer's disease compared to individuals in the top 10% of activity levels."* That's double the risk. Does their conclusion make you think twice about how active you are and how active you are going to become?

An article published in the *Canadian Family Physician* showed that there are multiple ways exercise protects the neurons of the brain. It strengthens the heart, protects the health of the arteries, and helps keep blood flowing to the neurons of the brain. The report showed that even in elderly people who already had cognitive impairment or dementia, their mental function improved with exercise. I point this out because in Mrs. Dell's case, this shows that exercise would have been beneficial even after she developed stage 2 MCI or even Alzheimer's dementia.

Here is the takeaway from this study. Regular physical activity, as compared with no exercise, was associated with a lower risk of cognitive impairment and Alzheimer's. *High levels of exercise reduced the incidence of Alzheimer's dementia by half.* The report showed that even in elderly people who already had cognitive impairment or dementia, mental function improved with exercise.

This same report examined the results of another study that found elderly people who did *less* than an hour of exercise daily, as compared with those who did *more* than an hour, had a *twofold increase in risk of cognitive decline.*

An *Archives of Neurology* article gave similar results, reporting that individuals who had symptoms of stage 2 Alzheimer's and who began exercising reduced their progression of symptoms when compared with those who did not exercise.

Strengthening the muscles of the heart helps it pump the maximum amount of blood with each beat. Only exercise builds the heart's strength and efficiency.

An article in *Neurology* reported a study that measured how much blood was pumped with each beat of the heart. Researchers studied 1,504 participants. None had any signs of a stroke or of impaired blood flow to the brain, and none showed any symptoms of Alzheimer's. The purpose of the study was to show that impaired heart muscle function is associated with a lower amount of blood to the brain and that this results in earlier signs of stage 1 Alzheimer's. MRI studies showed that the individuals with less heart strength, measured as cardiac index, showed shrinkage of certain parts of the brain even before symptoms of Alzheimer's were apparent. Their conclusion: *"Decreasing cardiac function is associated with accelerated brain aging."*

Work to *increase* your cardiac function—the strength of your heart. And remember, there is no medication that can strengthen your heart muscles. Only exercise can. Exercise is a large part of your plan for the prevention of even stage 1.

If you exercise, you will eat better. Exercise convinces your mind that you really mean business and gives you that extra boost in your eating lifestyle as well as your weight goals. So even brisk walking is going to have an additive effect on your overall prevention plan.

An article published in the *Annals of Internal Medicine* addressed the significance of exercise in people sixty-five and older. It is much better to begin your exercise program as young as possible, but exercise is important even at an older age.

Studies performed in middle age usually show individuals exercising much more intensely than studies of people over sixty-five. However, this report proves that even with very light exercise, there is a great protective cover against the progression of any dementia or Alzheimer's.

The study looked at whether people sixty-five and older who had normal mental function and exercised regularly were less likely to develop dementia over the coming years than those who did not exercise. The 1,740 participants all underwent routine mental testing and were followed for a six-year period.

The study also referred to other studies showing that the higher levels of physical fitness related to a greater tissue mass of the hippocampus, which you have learned plays a major role in memory. They suggested that the reason for this finding was because exercise improved blood flow to the hippocampus with increased oxygen and nutrient delivery.

The next part of their report caught my attention. The exercise assessment was unlike findings I had seen in so many other articles that pointed out that the more strenuous the exercise, the better protection of the arteries and the lower the risk of developing Alzheimer's. Most previous reports recommended thirty minutes a day for five to six days a week.

Researchers compared people who exercised more than three days a week with those who exercised less than three days a week. The duration of exercise was fifteen minutes per day. The type of exercise was not strenuous. The lightest type included walking, hiking, and stretching, while the more strenuous type included bicycling, swimming, and aerobics.

Those who exercised three or more times a week had a 32 percent reduction in their risk for Alzheimer's. Researchers pointed out that the results of this study were consistent with earlier studies showing that *even modest levels of physical exercise were associated with a delayed onset of Alzheimer's.*

"How long has she been asleep?" I asked Katy.

"Two hours. Just a nap. It's okay to wake her up."

"How are you doing, Mrs. Dell?" I had to watch her lips closely to see the words she was trying to express.

"Okay." That's all she said.

Then her eyes shut and her palm relaxed in mine. Asleep—again.

I realized the day was coming when she would look at me without knowing who I was. The battle would be lost. If she were to have an MRI or a PET scan, it would show the battlefield enlarged with few survivors and the fallen dead cells shrinking in the midst of the plaques. The day was coming when she would not know me. And even if she did, she wouldn't be able to express her thoughts. But my feelings for her would still be the same.

An interesting study done at Rush University Medical Center addressed the significance of exercise in older people. Researchers put a little device on the participants that recorded their average daily movements. The average age of the participants was eighty-two, and all were free from symptoms of Alzheimer's. Over the next four years, 10 percent of them developed Alzheimer's. The report concluded that *those who were in the least active 10 percent were twice as likely to develop Alzheimer's as those in the most active 10 percent.*

"A higher level of total daily physical activity is associated with a reduced risk of Alzheimer's Disease." That was the concluding statement following a study of more than seven hundred older individuals who didn't have any symptoms of Alzheimer's, as reported in the medical journal *Neurology*. The intensity of the physical activity was divided into tenths of percentiles. The exercise activities that were graded on intensity included everything from gardening to walking, calisthenics, bicycle riding, swimming, and water exercise. The study showed that a *person with high total daily physical activity*, which put them in the highest tenth percentile of exercisers, *was 2.3 times less likely to develop Alzheimer's than those who did the least exercise.*

A report in *Archives of Neurology* looked at a group of over four thousand people who were studied for a five-year follow-up period. The individuals were evaluated on the amount of exercise they did and placed into the three categories of low, moderate, and high levels of activity. Researchers concluded that *moderate and high levels of physical activity were associated with a 60 percent reduction in the risk for Alzheimer's.*

An article in the *Journal of Alzheimer's Disease* compared the intensity of the exercise to how well individuals did on mental tests and whether their MRI studies showed thicker or thinner brain mass. This study compared two groups of people who were sixty-five years or older. The individuals in the first group had no symptoms, while those in the second group were cognitively impaired. In other words, they showed symptoms of impairment related to mental function, reasoning, and memory. Researchers found that high levels of physical activity resulted in larger gray matter volumes in different lobes of the brain, including the hippocampus.

But what was really significant was that larger volumes were seen in both groups, the asymptomatic individuals as well as those who were cognitively impaired—those who had symptoms.

If all you can do is walk, will that help increase the size of your gray matter? A significant study looked into this question and was published in the journal *Neurology*. Researchers took 299 adults, mean age seventy-eight years old, who walked as their personal exercise routine and followed them for thirteen years. The group was divided into four tiers depending on how many blocks they walked. Researchers wanted to find out if walking had any effect on brain volume. They did MRIs to see if the brain matter in the people who didn't walk was different from the thickness of those who did. They also did mental testing on both to see if there was any difference in their scores. After following the participants for thirteen years, the conclusion was astonishing. Researchers found that *those who walked the greatest amounts had a greater amount of gray matter volume and also a reduced risk of cognitive impairment*. The area found to be the most positively affected was the hippocampus.

An interesting study called the Honolulu-Asia Aging Study looked at the relationship between walking and the mental problem of dementia. Researchers studied 2,257 men between the ages of seventy-one and ninety-three. *The men who walked less than one-quarter mile a day had almost twice the risk of developing dementia as the men who walked more than two miles a day.*

The takeaway from all these studies is this: if you don't have symptoms, exercise to prevent Alzheimer's; if you have symptoms, exercise to slow the progression of the disease. Do all you can do at any age, whether it is walking or high intensity exercise, to protect your brain.

I had believed walking was low in significance in terms of exercise. After reading the conclusions from these studies, never again will I look at older adults out walking and think they are wasting their time. No, I will now have the urge to go up and congratulate them for doing something great for their health.

Exercise:

- increases blood flow to the brain
- stimulates the growth of new neurons and synapses
- is associated with larger brain volume and less beta-amyloid
- reduces the risk of the heart and artery conditions that are associated with cognitive decline and dementia

I knew the day would arrive when tough decisions would need to be made concerning Mrs. Dell's last days. What if she couldn't swallow her food properly? What if she developed bedsores? Would she want her pneumonia treated? How would we decide?

One thing I was sure she would agree on. If it came to the point where she was heavily demented and for some reason her heart stopped beating, she would not want to be resuscitated. I heard it from friends, from patients, from almost anyone who ended up discussing what they would not want done to them if they were in a negative health state and the future was bleak. "Do not give me cardiac massage or place me on a respirator. Please make sure you don't let them do that to me. That's not the way I want to go out of this life."

It is still a difficult decision when the time comes and the doctors ask you about your spouse or child or friend. How would Mrs. Dell's ending be decided? Would her family all agree on what to do? Alzheimer's patients usually die of urinary infections or pneumonia. Would those be treated if Mrs. Dell developed them? Even if the doctors recommended not treating the infections and the family agreed to hold off on end-stage treatment, would Katy, even though she wasn't a member of the family, insist that everything possible be done to keep Mrs. Dell living?

Some Facts and Figures on Exercise and Alzheimer's

Here are some of the interesting numbers gleaned from the studies cited in this chapter.

1. A summary of a group of studies found that high levels of physical activity were associated with 38 percent lower risk of cognitive decline in older people without any symptoms of dementia.

2. There was a 45 percent reduced risk of Alzheimer's disease for those in the highest physical activity category compared to the lowest. Remember the article that encouraged me to write this book? Their study showed a 48 percent lower risk. Pretty close numbers for multiple studies to show.

3. Exercising at least twice a week at midlife was associated with a 52 percent reduced risk of dementia at ages 65–79.

Exercise and the Heart

Exercise strengthens the heart, lowers resting heart rate, lowers blood pressure, and lowers the oxygen demand of the heart muscle. All of these assist the heart in pumping more oxygen-rich blood to the brain.

Aerobic exercise, which is sustained exercise that increases the heart rate, is so important because it keeps the heart operating at peak performance. The stronger the heart, the easier it is to get blood throughout the body. The heart muscle is just like any other muscle. If it is forced to exercise, it becomes thicker and stronger.

I remember my first day of medical school like it was yesterday. "The heart is the single most important organ in your body except for your brain," our professor told us in anatomy lab. That anatomy class was exciting because I got to hold a human heart in my hand. I was able to look closely at the muscle makeup. I could see each artery lying on the surface of the muscle. When the professor spoke of the anterior descending coronary artery, I could see it, touch it. He then had us gather around the dissecting table. Several cadaver hearts were laid out on the slab, some with the muscle cut through and some with the arteries sliced open longitudinally to show blockages within the vessels. He wore a white lab coat, all three buttons neatly through each buttonhole. His head was freshly shaved, but you could tell he was mostly bald to begin with. And his shoes had been shined. His appearance was enough to make you pay attention to what he was about to say, but my eyes were fixed on what he held out toward us in his hands. In each hand, he held a human heart, both split open to show the main chamber.

I have never forgotten what he said next: "The heart in my right hand belonged to a gentleman who was what I call a couch potato. He was grossly overweight. He never exercised a day in his life. From his medical records, we know he was on numerous medications. As you can see, the wall of his left ventricle is only a few millimeters thick. His heart was a poor excuse for a pump, which he depended on every minute he was alive. Remember the thickness. Autopsy results revealed that he died from a massive heart attack—at the age of fifty-two.

"This man's heart is different," he said, indicating the heart in his left hand. "You see it is three to four times thicker than the first heart—much more muscle mass. It was strong right up to its last beat. He was trim, took good care of his body, didn't smoke, and was a frequent tennis player. This heart belonged to a sixty-one-year-old gentleman who died in an automobile accident. He was physiologically younger than the fifty-two-year-old couch potato. If you want to live younger, the only advice I can draw from these hearts is to be as active as you can be."

Next, he showed us a heart in which he had opened an artery longitudinally. He passed it around. The inside of the artery was as clean as a whistle. Then he passed around several hearts that had partial or complete blockages inside the arteries. He pointed out that most of the cadaver hearts he received from people who had died a non-accidental death had such blockages. He didn't know the actual cause of the blockages, but he knew they were the cause of the heart muscle not getting the oxygen it needed, resulting in the demise of that particular patient.

Then he made another statement I've never forgotten: "The ones with the least amount of blockage are the ones who lived longer."

When I think back to this, I have to remind myself of the statement in today's literature about Alzheimer's: what's good for the heart is good for the brain.

Exercise is the key to strengthening the muscles of your heart. Strengthening your heart muscle is similar to strengthening your biceps. The more you exercise it, the thicker and stronger the heart muscle gets. If you put a work force on the muscle, it responds by getting stronger. The greater the work force, the more times it will beat per minute during that work force. When you die, you want the pathologist to look at your heart and remark how thick and strong the muscle looks.

Your Personal Exercise Plan

I would like to give you a simple plan for strengthening the muscles in your heart so that it can sustain the amount of blood for your brain to function at peak performance.

Jogging is one of the best ways to strengthen your heart because it keeps your heart at an elevated sustained heart rate for a specific period of time. An article in the *Archives of Internal Medicine* points this out. The study, which began in 1976, involved twenty thousand men and women. Their ages ranged from twenty to ninety-three. The study compared a subgroup of joggers to a subgroup of non-joggers. The difference they found between the two groups is significant. The joggers ran for thirty minutes a day, two to five days a week.

There was a significant increase in life expectancy for the group that jogged. The study showed that the risk of death was reduced by 44 percent in the jogging group. The data showed that *jogging was linked with an added 6.2 years of life expectancy in men and 5.6 years in women.* The better the blood supply to your heart, the better the blood supply will be to your brain.

The question to ask is, why does jogging extend your life? The most significant reason that exercise such as jogging extends your life is that it strengthens your heart muscle. I encourage you to perform some type of aerobic exercise thirty minutes a day, six days a week. Not only will you extend your life expectancy, but you will also have quality time during each of those extra years. The first thing to do is commit to a plan. Then stick with it.

Aerobic Exercise Plan

Let's begin with a plan to get you moving if exercise is new for you. If you cannot jog yet, simply begin with a thirty-minute walk at a steady pace, six days a week. The following week, move to a faster walk, and eventually to a brisk walk. Committing to a thirty-minute walk may be the most significant decision you ever make. You will have "begun." Do what you can do and keep working to improve.

It doesn't matter where you are on your exercise continuum: just commit to starting a thirty-minute program. Remember, there is much more to it than just how vigorous the exercise is. Exercising sends a message to your brain about your commitment to eat the proper foods and get to your ideal weight. If exercise is new for you, here is a plan to get you started. It will help you strengthen your heart so it can supply the amount of blood your brain needs to function at peak performance.

Week 1, Days 1–6	30 minutes walking
Week 2, Days 1–3	2 minutes jogging, 28 minutes walking
Week 2, Days 4–6	3 minutes jogging, 27 minutes walking
Week 3, Days 1–3	4 minutes jogging, 26 minutes walking
Week 3, Days 4–6	5 minutes jogging, 25 minutes walking
Week 4, Days 1–3	6 minutes jogging, 24 minutes walking

Week 4, Days 4–6	7 minutes jogging, 23 minutes walking
Week 5, Days 1–3	8 minutes jogging, 22 minutes walking
Week 5, Days 4–6	9 minutes jogging, 21 minutes walking
Week 6, Days 1–3	10 minutes jogging, 20 minutes walking
Week 6, Days 4–6	12 minutes jogging, 18 minutes walking
Week 7, Days 1–3	14 minutes jogging, 16 minutes walking
Week 7, Days 4–6	16 minutes jogging, 14 minutes walking
Week 8, Days 1–3	18 minutes jogging, 12 minutes walking
Week 8, Days 4–6	20 minutes jogging, 10 minutes walking
Week 9, Days 1–3	22 minutes jogging, 8 minutes walking
Week 9, Days 4–6	24 minutes jogging, 6 minutes walking
Week 10, Days 1–3	26 minutes jogging, 4 minutes walking
Week 10, Days 4–6	28 minutes jogging, 2 minutes walking
Week 11, Days 1–6	30 minutes jogging

After you can jog for thirty consecutive minutes, focus on increasing your pace. Set your own personal goals. But above all else, get off the couch and get started.

16

Bonus Lifestyle Choices

Defeating Dementia by Staying Mentally and Socially Active

Mrs. Dell lay in the bed and stared straight ahead most of the time or kept her eyes closed. She couldn't turn herself over. Katy and the other caregivers rolled her every two hours, side to side, and placed small pillows to balance her body. She wore a diaper constantly.

There were times when Katy and the other caregivers thought Mrs. Dell responded to them. She would open one or both eyes when they spoke to her. "She can tell it's me," Katy would remind me repeatedly. "She knows my voice and my laugh. I sing to her all the time."

Katy was the one who used to take Mrs. Dell to the doctor for her routine follow-ups. One day I asked Katy if she had ever talked to the doctor about taking Mrs. Dell off the medicine.

"There could be side effects that may be bad. It may be simpler for her not to take it and for you not to give it," I said. "I'm not an expert concerning Alzheimer's, but I don't think it is helping her situation at this time, and I just wondered if her doctor ever mentioned stopping some of the pills or changing them."

"No, sir. And even if the doctor considered taking her off her medicine, I would feel terrible if we took her off and she got worse."

Before we finish our journey, let's look at additional things you can do to reduce your risk of Alzheimer's. Staying mentally and socially active has many positive benefits for your brain in addition to adding fun to your years.

PET scans show that mental activities that stimulate the thinking process during midlife are associated with reduced beta-amyloid in the brain in late life. Examples include keeping up with current events, reading, playing games, and studying items that are of interest to you. Take a course at a local college. Take up a new hobby. Keep your brain working.

Scientists don't know exactly how keeping your mind active protects you against beta-amyloid formation. One possibility makes sense but hasn't been proven. Individuals who participate in a variety of mentally stimulating activities during their lives may develop a more proficient communication between neurons and synapses that results in less beta-amyloid deposition. It is called the "use it or lose it" concept or the "cognitive stimulation lifestyle."

Social activity has also been shown to reduce the risk of dementia. In a study of 1,772 people who were over sixty-five, *those who were the most active from a social aspect had a 38 percent lower risk of developing dementia than the individuals who did not participate in such activities.* Examples of their activities included visiting with friends or entertaining in their homes. Some volunteered in their communities with clubs and church organizations. Others played games socially. Such reports encourage us all to stay socially active rather than becoming recluses.

I sat beside her bed. She didn't talk anymore. She tried. She was merely a shadow of what she used to be. But my memory of her was as bright as the noonday sun. When I asked her a question, sometimes she moved her mouth, but she couldn't get her lips coordinated to make a word come out. I knew she heard me because her attempts to speak always immediately followed my questions to her. *Should I not ask her any more questions?* I wondered.

Did she understand my questions? If she could answer, would what she was trying to say make sense?

It would be so terrible to be lying there—and listening and hearing—and understanding exactly what was being said or asked, and to know exactly how you wanted to answer, know each and every word you wanted to say—yet not be able to say them.

The Last Leaf

It was one of my last visits with Mrs. Dell. She mostly slept. After Mr. Dell died, she still slept in the queen-sized bed. Then she was moved to a single bed for easier entrance and exit, followed by a hospital bed in the bedroom, and then a specialized bed in the living room with an air mattress that changed inflation areas to prevent bedsores.

It was getting more difficult to get her attention. Too much of Mrs. Dell had been taken away.

I tried to communicate with her. I talked to her because I believed she could hear me. I wanted to believe she understood me. I asked her how she was feeling, if she got enough sleep last night. I wondered if she wanted something to drink. To eat. Just to nibble on. She just lay there, sometimes with her eyes open and other times closed. Then occasionally she raised her eyelids when I asked a question. I wondered, *Is she really there? Or am I just kidding myself?*

I sensed I was nearing my last visit. I was pretty certain she wouldn't know who I was. Were any neurons working well enough for her to realize I was there? Had there been too many battles with the plaques and the tangles and the mini-strokes within her mind that there were now no survivors? Or did a group of neurons remain healthy enough for her to recognize me, hear what I was saying, even if she couldn't respond to my questions? I couldn't see what was happening. I could only imagine. So much of Alzheimer's remains in the dark.

I stood on the right side of her bed and watched her. Her silver hair, brushed to perfection by Katy, was resting on the pillow. For some reason, she looked different to me. The skin on her face looked thinner and ghostly white. Her lips were as thin as two pieces of paper, one laid on top of the other.

Mrs. Dell stared straight at the ceiling for a few minutes and then closed her eyes. I decided to speak to her—but nothing changed. I repeated the same thing again louder and then a third time. She reopened her eyes but didn't look at me. Only at the ceiling.

I realized that being alive and living are worlds apart. Mrs. Dell was alive but not really living. The light was getting dimmer. Her mind was filling with darkness. I wondered how many more tomorrows she had. How many leaves were yet dangling?

If only I knew what was happening in Mrs. Dell's mind. There was no test to determine whether she could understand what I was saying to her. It would have been great to know she knew each time I visited her, spoke to her, and told her how much I loved her. It would have been great to know she understood she was still cared for. It would have been great to know she still enjoyed hearing Katy sing to her.

I remembered a patient who experienced a stroke and was in the hospital. I spoke to him and asked him questions but received no response. He eventually recovered and told me later that he could understand what I was saying to him. He remembered the questions I had asked. He said the answers were in his brain, but he couldn't make himself communicate with me. His thoughts seemed packed in a closed container, and he couldn't find the key to open the box to get them out. He told me how hard he had tried to talk to me, but he just couldn't make it happen. He just lay there and stared at the ceiling—like Mrs. Dell was doing. But he knew what was going on. I wondered if Mrs. Dell's mind was doing the same.

Three months earlier when I picked up her wrist to lay her hand in mine, she barely had the strength to hold up her hand. Back then she at least could squeeze my thumb. But this time as I lifted her arm with my hand, it was almost completely limp. She couldn't grasp my thumb. I gently touched the palm of her hand with mine. No response. Her hand remained limp.

I knew this day would come. It was difficult for me to accept that the battle was finally lost.

I don't know why the thought came to me, but I bent toward her ear and fairly loudly told her, "Mrs. Dell, if you stick your tongue out at me, you will get a spanking." Her eyelids didn't even quiver.

I spoke a little louder. "Mrs. Dell, if you stick your tongue out at me, you will get a spanking." There were several people in the room, and we all watched to see if there would be any kind of response. I held her limp hand in mine. I kept my thoughts to myself.

But I knew it was over.

"Look, look," Katy whispered excitedly, pointing to Mrs. Dell's lips. "Look at her lips." We all looked and watched both lips begin to quiver. On the left side of her mouth, the part of the upper lip that was hiding the lower lifted slightly.

I bent closer to evaluate what I had just given up on, and what I saw I could not believe. In the very center, between her lips, was the very tip of a minute protrusion. It looked like a little red dot. I was shocked to realize what it was. It was the tip of her tongue.

"Look, look!" This time Katy was yelling and clapping her hands and laughing loudly.

As we all watched, her tongue began to protrude more and more until her mouth was wide open. I could even see the back of her throat as she slowly but forcefully pushed her entire tongue forward until it ended up lying flat, completely covering her lower lip.

I couldn't believe it, but it was real. Mrs. Dell was still alive and aware. I realized she had not yet gone.

She heard me.

She understood me.

Her defiant action with her tongue proved it.

I looked down at her lying flat in bed. My throat tightened as I attempted to swallow, but I couldn't. She was still fighting the battle.

All I could do was gently place my arms around her shoulders as I kissed her forehead. I held her for a long time before reminding her, "We all love you, Mrs. Dell, and I will never let anyone spank you."

Several weeks later, Katy called the ambulance to take Mrs. Dell to the hospital because she couldn't swallow her medicine. At the hospital, she was found to have a urinary tract infection, and her esophagus was not functioning normally. She was given IV fluids with antibiotics for her urinary tract infection, but she never regained the ability to swallow. After four days, the doctors told her family a decision had to be made. Either a small feeding tube would have to be inserted into her nose and down to her stomach to furnish food and water, or she would need to be transferred to hospice for comfort care only. If her swallowing ability didn't return, the feeding tube would need to be replaced with a feeding tube inserted through her abdomen and into her stomach.

A feeding tube or hospice. That was the choice.

Katy was toward the back of the room, but she called out the one question on her mind: "What are the chances she will be able to swallow again?"

The doctor replied quickly and matter-of-factly, "The odds are—she won't regain the ability to swallow."

"But if you don't put in a tube and she goes to hospice and you don't feed her and give her water, she's going to get so thirsty and hungry. That would be terrible." Katy's eyes traveled from the doctor to me, and she asked, "What would you do if you had to make the decision?"

I explained to Katy and the family what I remembered from the first time in my medical career when a similar question had been asked. I began my remembrance. "I was in surgical training and attending a meeting to decide what treatment was the most appropriate for a cancer patient. The patient had had lung cancer removed. But the cancer had spread to the liver, the brain, and the opposite lung.

"The oncologist went first. She explained that the patient should undergo chemotherapy first, before any radiation. Her drugs would target the tumor cells wherever they were hiding. There would be three drugs, one of them a trial drug. It was not known whether this particular drug would be effective or what the side effects would be.

"Next the radiation therapy doctor spoke. He could knock out the cancer in the remaining lung, but the radiation would have some effect on the patient's breathing."

Katy and everyone in the room were giving me their full attention as I finished my recollection. "After the oncologist and the radiologist finished their recommendations, my surgery professor rose from his seat and made one statement that concluded the discussion. He looked around the room and said, 'There comes a time when the best treatment for certain patients is a fishing pole and a tall glass of tea.' He sat back down, and there was quietness until the oncologist replied that she wholeheartedly agreed. She would recommend, rather than giving him chemotherapy, giving him whatever was needed to keep him comfortable. The radiation therapy doctor also agreed to comfort measures."

I said no more. I knew my conclusion was right, and I hoped the family and Katy would understand that the best path for Mrs. Dell was the one that would keep her comfortable.

The decision was made not to put her through the trauma of having a tube in her nose and going through an operation and making her spend the remainder of her life suffering.

The hospice caregivers explained that they would keep her mouth moist and they would give her IV morphine to control any discomfort she might have.

I went to see her in hospice. While she lay in bed with her eyes closed, her children and her grandchildren talked to her, sang her favorite songs to her, and prayed with her. Mrs. Dell passed away, a serene death, several days later. She spent her last days in peaceful rest—with her fishing pole and a tall glass of tea by her side.

And with a gentle breeze, the last leaf fell.

Epilogue

Mr. Dell was a good husband to the end. But about two years before he died, he received a knee replacement and developed complications that immobilized him for several months. He developed an infection, couldn't walk or get around except via a wheelchair, and was placed in a rest home. We weren't certain he would survive such serious complications.

Mr. Dell's daughter asked if I would do her a very personal favor. "Would you go talk with my father to see if he's a Christian? I know he has been a very good man. I know he went to church with my mother on a regular basis. But what I don't know is whether he ever accepted Jesus as his Savior for eternity. And I want to be sure."

I knew Mr. Dell quite well. He had such a kind heart for others. If doing good deeds could get you into heaven, Mr. Dell would make it. But I knew that wasn't the answer his daughter was looking for. One of his coworkers from the courthouse shared an insightful story with me. He was the magistrate court constable for the county. Part of Mr. Dell's job was to present summonses to people who had not paid their rent for an extended period of time. After an additional specified period of time, some might have to be evicted from their homes if a court so ordered. Then Mr. Dell would drive to the home, knock on the door, and explain to the occupants they would have to leave.

He had told me before that this was the worst part of his job. He hated to evict anyone from their home, even if it was a court order. But that was his job.

Mr. Dell's coworker told me the story of Mr. Dell going out into the county to evict a lady and her three children. The mother knew the time was coming. She hadn't paid any rent in over five months. What furniture she owned would be placed outside the house, the door would be shut and locked, and she would not be able to go back inside. Ever.

Mr. Dell left behind the two men who accompanied him in the eviction to remove all the furniture. They completed their job and locked the doors to the house with special locks.

The family left to go to a friend's house for the remainder of the day and evening. The furniture remained in the yard.

Shortly after lunch, a rain cloud appeared. Mr. Dell received word that a thunderstorm was approaching the area. He drove his truck home to where he stored some tarpaulin rain covers. He loaded them into the back of his truck, drove back to the house in the country, and covered all the exposed furniture with the tarps. The rains came, but the furniture was protected.

Mr. Dell himself shared this story with me: "I was walking down the sidewalk in front of the courthouse one day when a man crossing the street smiled, waved his arm, and asked me how I was doing." Mr. Dell started smiling as he continued his story. "I thought the man was probably a friend but couldn't quite place him. I asked him to remind me who he was." Mr. Dell laughed softly as he quoted the man's answer: "'Don't you remember me? I'm the fella you evicted out on Highway 41 about a year ago. You have a good day, Mr. Dell.'

"You would have thought we were the best of friends," Mr. Dell said to me.

I knew Mr. Dell's heart, but just because you have a kind heart doesn't mean you will spend eternity with God. That is why his daughter wanted me to speak to him. She knew what a gentle and kind man he was. She knew his heart. But she didn't know for certain if he had a faith in Jesus that would give him eternal life in heaven.

I found Mr. Dell lying in bed reading the local paper as I entered his room. He promptly folded it and laid it aside. "Hey, Mr. Dell. How are you feeling today?"

He explained it was a good day and thought his infection was improving. "I think I will get out of here one of these days." He laughed.

We carried on a fairly routine conversation as I tried to figure out exactly how to ask him about his faith. I decided to begin with a question.

"Did I ever tell you about discussions I had with my post-op cancer patients in the follow-up exams in my office? What I would ask them about their future?" I knew he had no idea where I was headed. As he slightly shook his head no, I continued.

"Every patient who gets a cancer diagnosis has to at least think about what is going to happen to them when they die. Whether it is from their cancer or another disease, the thought of death has to enter their minds."

Mr. Dell kept his eyes focused on mine.

"I asked them if they would like to discuss eternity. I never wanted to force my conversation on them, so I would always ask. Every one of them responded that they would like such a discussion.

"I would then turn toward the examining room door and point to it, explaining that if they were to die right now and that was the door into heaven, and they knocked on the door—what one thing could they say that would guarantee them getting into heaven?

"Probably two-thirds of them responded that they hoped they had done more good than bad, and, that is what they would tell the gatekeeper." I looked at him as he kept his focus on me.

"Your daughter asked me to ask you this same question."

His eyebrows rose slightly. As if he didn't know why she would wonder such a thing. I waited for his response.

"Well, I do think I have done more good than bad through-out my life." His eyes moved away from me and toward the beauty of the day outside the window of his first-floor room. He continued, "But I know that is not what counts on that day. I know I have sinned at times in my life. I realize I haven't been a perfect man." He quickly cut his eyes back directly to mine as he made his next statement. "And neither have you." Back to the window now. "But I also believe that God sent his Son, Jesus, to die for my sins. And yours also. It has been many, many years ago that I realized this and I accepted that belief as a gift. I asked Jesus to come into my heart that day. I turned it all over to him. That's where my faith is." Mr. Dell now looked back at me with a slight smile. "Don't you worry—I'm going to end up in heaven."

"Mr. Dell, that is the perfect answer." I reached over the side of the bed and lightly placed my hand on his shoulder. "What you just said is similar to the verse I tell the patients who do not know the correct answer. This verse explains it better than I ever could. It is basically what you have just answered. It says: 'Jesus answered, "I am the way and the truth and the life. No one comes to the Father except through me."'"

Mr. Dell's smile broadened. "I agree. And you can tell her what I said about knocking on the door to heaven. You can give her that assurance about her dad. I probably should have told her before . . . But I always assumed she knew."

He folded his hands over his chest as he relaxed his head on the pillow and closed his eyes to rest.

Conclusion

The time of commitment has come. You need to commit to do all you can to prevent the onset of the most frightening disease as you age. Make a life-changing decision to prevent having to travel the most dreaded path you and your loved ones could ever travel. The changes you make now will affect the quality of your life from this day on. Whether you are thirty or seventy, you can do things that will make you younger physiologically, even as you age chronologically, and at the same time will ward off dementia.

It's not a difficult decision. You now know medically what goes on in the brain as Alzheimer's develops. It is my hope that with this new knowledge you will find it easier to eat a healthy diet, get to your ideal weight, and make exercise a way of life.

The changes you make will also affect your loved ones. Mrs. Dell wasn't the only one affected by Alzheimer's. Mr. Dell, her children, and her grandchildren all suffered. Her friends and caregivers sacrificed for her. Alzheimer's is an enemy that doesn't attack only a single individual. It assaults the multitude of people who have to change their thoughts and actions and finances in order to care for a loved one who suffers for so long.

I encourage you to consider the direction you are now traveling and realize that the path you are on determines your future. It would give me the greatest satisfaction to know that the time we've spent together in this book has helped you make a decisive change that will affect the remainder of your life.

Remember, with commitment comes hope for the future.

References

Journals

Acta Neurologica Scandinavica: Supplementum
"Cholesterol as a Risk Factor for Alzheimer's Disease—Epidemiological Evidence." 185 (2006): 50–57.

Acta Neuropathologica
"The Overlap between Neurodegenerative and Vascular Factors in the Pathogenesis of Dementia." 120 (2010): 287–96.

Acta Psychiatrica Scandinavica
"Trends in Prevalence of Alzheimer's Disease and Vascular Dementia in a Japanese Community: The Hisayama Study." 122 (2010): 319–25.

Advances in Nutrition
"ω-3 Fatty Acids in the Prevention of Cognitive Decline in Humans." 4 (2013): 672–76.

Age and Aging
"Smoking, Hypercholesterolaemia, and Hypertension as Risk Factors for Cognitive Impairment in Older Adults." 42 (2013): 306–11.

Aging

"Heart Disease and Vascular Risk Factors in the Cognitively Impaired Elderly: Implications for Alzheimer's Dementia." 13 (2001): 231–39.

Aging and Mental Health

"Is Physical Activity a Potential Preventive Factor for Vascular Dementia? A Systematic Review." 14 (2010): 386–95.

Aging Research Reviews

"Blood Pressure and the Risk for Dementia: A Double-Edged Sword." 8 (2009): 61–70.

"Demonstrating the Case that AD Is a Vascular Disease: Epidemiologic Evidence." 1 (2002): 61–77.

"Vascular Risk Factor Detection and Control May Prevent Alzheimer's Disease." 9 (2010): 218–25.

Alzheimer Disease and Associated Disorders

"Prevention of Dementia by Intensive Vascular Care (PreDIVA): A Cluster-Randomized Trial in Progress." 23 (2009): 198–204.

"Vascular Risk Factors for Incident Alzheimer Disease and Vascular Dementia: The Cache County Study." 20 (2006): 93–100.

Alzheimer's and Dementia

"Atherosclerosis Risk in Communities Study Brain MRI Study. Fourteen-Year Longitudinal Study of Vascular Risk Factors, APOE Genotype, and Cognition: The ARIC MRI Study." 5 (2009): 207–14.

"Effects of n-3 Fatty Acids on Cognitive Decline: A Randomized, Double-Blind, Placebo-Controlled Trial in Stable Myocardial Infarction Patients." 8 (2012): 278–87.

"The Finnish Geriatric Intervention Study to Prevent Cognitive Impairment and Disability (FINGER): Study Design and Progress." 9 (2013): 657–65.

"Mediterranean Diet, Micronutrients and Macronutrients, and MRI Measures of Cortical Thickness." 23 (2016): S1552–5260(16)32661–69.

"MIND Diet Associated with Reduced Incidence of Alzheimer's Disease." 11 (2015): 1007–14.

"Toward Defining the Preclinical Stages of Alzheimer's Disease: Recommendations from the National Institute on Aging–Alzheimer's Association Workgroups on Diagnostic Guidelines for Alzheimer's Disease." 7 (2011): 280–92.

"2014 Alzheimer's Disease Facts and Figures." 10 (2014): 47–92.

"2012 Alzheimer's Disease Facts and Figures." 8 (2012): 131–68.

"Vascular Contributions to Cognitive Impairment and Dementia Including Alzheimer's Disease." 11 (2015): 710–17.

Alzheimer's Research and Therapy

"Dementia Prevention: Current Epidemiological Evidence and Future Perspective." 4 (2012): 6.

American Journal of Clinical Nutrition

"Accruing Evidence on Benefits of Adherence to the Mediterranean Diet on Health: An Updated Systematic Review and Meta-analysis." 92 (2010): 1189–96.

"Adherence to a Mediterranean-Type Dietary Pattern and Cognitive Decline in a Community Population." 93 (2011): 601–7.

"Brain Atrophy in Cognitively Impaired Elderly: The Importance of Long-Chain ω-3 Fatty Acids and B Vitamin Status in a Randomized Controlled Trial." 102 (2015): 215–21.

American Journal of Geriatric Pharmacotherapy

"Cardiovascular Risk Factors and Dementia." 6 (2008): 100–118.

American Neurological Association

"Subcortical Infarcts, Alzheimer's Disease Pathology, and Memory Function in Older Persons." 62 (2007): 59–66.

Annals of Epidemiology

"Cross-Sectional and Longitudinal Changes in Total and High-Density Lipoprotein Cholesterol Levels over a Twenty-Year Period in Elderly Men: The Honolulu Heart Program." 7 (1997): 417–24.

Annals of Internal Medicine

"Diabetes in Midlife and Cognitive Change over Twenty Years: A Cohort Study." 161 (2014): 785–93.

"Exercise in People Age 65 Years and Older Is Associated with Lower Risk for Dementia." 144 (2006): 120.

"Exercise Is Associated with Reduced Risk for Incident Dementia among Persons 65 Years of Age and Older." 144 (2006): 73–81.

"National Institutes of Health State-of-the-Science Conference Statement: Preventing Alzheimer Disease and Cognitive Decline." 153 (2010): 176–81.

Annals of Neurology

"Apolipoprotein E and Cognitive Change in an Elderly Population." 40 (1996): 55–66.

"Atherosclerosis, Dementia, and Alzheimer Disease in the Baltimore Longitudinal Study of Aging Cohort." 68 (2010): 231–40.

"Cerebral Hypoperfusion and Clinical Onset of Dementia: The Rotterdam Study." 57 (2005): 789–94.

"Dietary Fat Intake and the Risk of Incident Dementia in the Rotterdam Study." 42 (1997): 776–82.

"Mediterranean Diet and Risk for Alzheimer's Disease." 59 (2006): 912–21.

Annals of the New York Academy of Sciences

"Cholesterol in Alzheimer's Disease and Tauopathy." 977 (2002): 367–75.

"Vascular Involvement in Cognitive Decline and Dementia: Epidemiologic Evidence from the Rotterdam Study and the Rotterdam Scan Study." 903 (2000): 457–65.

Archives of Internal Medicine

"An Eighteen-Year Follow-up of Overweight and Risk of Alzheimer Disease." 163 (2003): 1524–28.

"A Prospective Study of Physical Activity and Cognitive Decline in Elderly Women: Women Who Walk." 161 (2001): 1703–8.

Archives of Neurology

"Antihypertensive Medication Use and Incident Alzheimer Disease: The Cache County Study." 63 (2006): 686–92.

"Association of Higher Levels of High-Density Lipoprotein Cholesterol in Elderly Individuals and Lower Risk of Late-Onset Alzheimer Disease." 67 (2010): 1491–97.

"Consumption of Fish and n-3 Fatty Acids and Risk of Incident Alzheimer Disease." 60 (2003): 940–46.

"Contribution of Vascular Risk Factors to the Progression in Alzheimer Disease." 66 (2009): 343–48.

"Dietary Fats and the Risk of Incident Alzheimer Disease." 60 (2003): 194–200.

"Effects of Aerobic Exercise on Mild Cognitive Impairment: A Controlled Trial." 67 (2010): 71–79.

"Fish Consumption and Cognitive Decline with Age in a Large Community Study." 62 (2005): 1849–53.

"Mediterranean Diet, Alzheimer Disease, and Vascular Mediation." 63 (2006): 1709–17.

"Mediterranean Diet and Mild Cognitive Impairment." 66 (2009): 216–25.

"Midlife and Late-Life Obesity and the Risk of Dementia: Cardiovascular Health Study." 66 (2009): 336–42.

"Physical Activity and Risk of Cognitive Impairment and Dementia in Elderly Persons." 58 (2001): 498–504.

"Poststroke Dementia: Influence of Hippocampal Atrophy." 60 (2003): 585–90.

"Promising Strategies for the Prevention of Dementia." 66 (2009): 1210–15.

"The Role of Metabolic Disorders in Alzheimer Disease and Vascular Dementia: Two Roads Converged." 66 (2009): 300–305.

"Statin Use and the Risk of Incident Dementia: The Cardiovascular Health Study." 62 (2005): 1047–51.

"Stroke and the Risk of Alzheimer Disease." 60 (2003): 1707–12.

"Twenty-Six-Year Change in Total Cholesterol Levels and Incident Dementia: The Honolulu-Asia Aging Study." 64 (2007): 103–7.

Arteriosclerosis, Thrombosis, and Vascular Biology
"Brain Cholesterol: Long Secret Life behind a Barrier." 24 (2004): 806–15.

Biochemical and Biophysical Research Communications
"Elevated Low-Density Lipoprotein in Alzheimer's Disease Correlates with Brain Abeta 1–42 Levels." 252 (1998): 711–15.

Biochemical Pharmacology
"Future Directions in Alzheimer's Disease from Risk Factors to Prevention." 88 (2014): 661–70.

Biological Psychiatry
"Meta-analysis of Alzheimer's Disease Risk with Obesity, Diabetes, and Related Disorders." 67 (2010): 505–12.

Biomarkers in Medicine
"Alzheimer's Prevention Initiative: A Proposal to Evaluate Presymptomatic Treatments as Quickly as Possible." 4 (2010): 3–14.

BMC Geriatrics
"Lipoprotein Profile in Older Patients with Vascular Dementia and Alzheimer's Disease." 1 (2001): 5.

BMC Neurology
"Framingham Stroke Risk Profile and Poor Cognitive Function: A Population-Based Study." 8 (2008): 12.
"Promotion of the Mind through Exercise (PROMoTE): A Proof-of-Concept Randomized Controlled Trial of Aerobic Exercise Training in Older Adults with Vascular Cognitive Impairment." 10 (2010): 14.

BMC Psychiatry
"Protocol for a Randomized Controlled Trial Evaluating the Effect of Physical Activity on Delaying the Progression of White Matter Changes on MRI in Older Adults with Memory Complaints and Mild Cognitive Impairment: The AIBL Active Trial." 12 (2012): 167.

Brain

"Profiles of Neuropsychological Impairment in Autopsy-Defined Alzheimer's Disease and Cerebrovascular Disease." 130 (2007): 731–39.

British Medical Journal

"Midlife Vascular Risk Factors and Alzheimer's Disease in Later Life: Longitudinal, Population Based Study." 322 (2001): 1447–51.

"Obesity in Middle Age and Future Risk of Dementia: A Twenty-Seven-Year Longitudinal Population Based Study." 330 (2005): 1360.

Canadian Family Physician

"Prevention of Alzheimer Disease: Encouraging Evidence." 52 (2006): 200–207.

Cell Metabolism

"Hypertension and Cerebrovascular Dysfunction." 7 (2008): 476–84.

Circulation

"Diet and Lifestyle Recommendations Revision 2006: A Scientific Statement from the American Heart Association Nutrition Committee." 114 (2006): 82–96.

"Physical Activity and Public Health in Older Adults: Recommendation from the American College of Sports Medicine and the American Heart Association." 116 (2007): 1094–105.

Clinical Interventions in Aging

"Omega-3 Fatty Acids: Potential Role in the Management of Early Alzheimer's Disease." 5 (2010): 45–61.

Clinical Science

"The Vascular Contribution to Alzheimer's Disease." 119 (2010): 407–21.

CNS Drugs

"Prevention Studies in Alzheimer's Disease: Progress towards the Development of New Therapeutics." 29 (2015): 519–28.

Current Alzheimer Research

"Cholesterol and LDL Relate to Neuritic Plaques and to APOE4 Presence but Not to Neurofibrillary Tangles." 8 (2011): 303–12.

"Dietary Omega-3 Polyunsaturated Fatty Acids and Alzheimer's Disease: Interaction with Apolipoprotein E Genotype." 8 (2011): 479–91.

"Overview and Findings from the Rush Memory and Aging Project." 9 (2012): 646–63.

"Relation of Obesity to Cognitive Function: Importance of Central Obesity and Synergistic Influence of Concomitant Hypertension: The Framingham Heart Study." 4 (2007): 111–16.

Current Atherosclerosis Reports

"Cardiovascular Risk Factors and Alzheimer's Disease." 6 (2004): 261–66.

Dementia and Geriatric Cognitive Disorders

"Elevated Serum Total and LDL Cholesterol in Very Old Patients with Alzheimer's Disease." 12 (2001): 138–45.

"Rethinking the Dementia Diagnoses in a Population-Based Study: What Is Alzheimer's Disease and What Is Vascular Dementia? A Study from the Kungsholmen Project." 22 (2006): 244–49.

Epidemiologic Reviews

"Type 2 Diabetes as a Risk Factor for Alzheimer's Disease: The Confounders, Interactions, and Neuropathology Associated with This Relationship." 35 (2013): 152–60.

Epidemiology

"Mediterranean Diet, Cognitive Function, and Dementia: A Systematic Review." 24 (2013): 479–89.

European Geriatric Medicine

"Exercise, Fitness, and Cognition: A Randomised Controlled Trial in Older Individuals: The DR's EXTRA Study." 1 (2010): 266–72.

European Journal of Clinical Nutrition

"Dietary Fat Intake in Relation to Cognitive Change in High-Risk Women with Cardiovascular Disease or Vascular Factors." 64 (2010): 1134–40.

European Journal of Neurology

"Cause of Death in Patients with Dementia Disorders." 16 (2009): 488–92.

European Journal of Pharmacology

"Adiposity, Hyperinsulinemia, Diabetes, and Alzheimer's Disease: An Epidemiological Perspective." 585 (2008): 119–29.

Experimental Gerontology

"Chronic Mild Cerebrovascular Dysfunction as a Cause for Alzheimer's Disease?" 46 (2011): 225–32.

Expert Review of Neurotherapeutics

"Diet and Alzheimer's Disease Risk Factors or Prevention: The Current Evidence." 11 (2011): 677–708.

Focus on Healthy Aging

"Alzheimer's Disease: Advances in Prevention and Treatment." souforum. com/2016/11/18/3-who-is-at-risk-for-alzheimers-disease.

Finnish Cardiovascular Risk Factors, Aging, and Incidence of Dementia

"Obesity and Vascular Risk Factors at Midlife and the Risk of Dementia and Alzheimer's Disease." 62 (2005): 1556–60.

Frontiers in Nutrition

"Adherence to a Mediterranean-Style Diet and Effects on Cognition in Adults: A Qualitative Evaluation and Systematic Review of Longitudinal and Prospective Trials." 3 (2016): 22.

Healthy Aging Research

"Translation of Low-Risk Dementia-Associated Interventions into Practice—a Call to Action." 4 (2015): 1–9.

Hippocampus

"Low-Intensity Daily Walking Activity Is Associated with Hippocampal Volume in Older Adults." 25 (2015): 605–15.

Hypertension

"Blood Pressure Trajectories from Midlife to Late Life in Relation to Dementia in Women Followed for Thirty-Seven Years." 59 (2012): 796–801.

"Effects of the Dietary Approaches to Stop Hypertension: Diet, Exercise, and Caloric Restriction on Neurocognition in Overweight Adults with High Blood Pressure." 55 (2010): 1331–38.

"Hypertension Is Related to Cognitive Impairment: A Twenty-Year Follow-up of 999 Men." 31 (1998): 780–86.

"Midlife Blood Pressure, Plasma β-Amyloid, and the Risk for Alzheimer Disease: The Honolulu-Asia Aging Study." 59 (2012): 780–86.

International Journal of Obesity

"Lower Cognitive Function in the Presence of Obesity and Hypertension: the Framingham Heart Study." 27 (2003): 260–68.

Journal of Alzheimer's Disease

"Alzheimer's Prevention Initiative: A Plan to Accelerate the Evaluation of Presymptomatic Treatments." 26 (2011): 321–29.

"Atherosclerosis in the Evolution of Alzheimer's Disease: Can Treatment Reduce Cognitive Decline?" 20 (2010): 893–901.

"Brain Cholesterol Metabolism, Oxysterols, and Dementia." 33 (2013): 891–911.

"Can the Treatment of Vascular Risk Factors Slow Cognitive Decline in Alzheimer's Disease Patients?" 32 (2012): 765–72.

"Is There a Characteristic Lipid Profile in Alzheimer's Disease?" 6 (2004): 585–89, 673–81.

"Longitudinal Relationships between Caloric Expenditure and Gray Matter in the Cardiovascular Health Study." 52 (2016): 719–29.

"Midlife Vascular Risk Factors and Alzheimer's Disease: Evidence from Epidemiological Studies." 32 (2012): 531–40.

"Polyunsaturated Fatty Acids and Reduced Odds of MCI: The Mayo Clinic Study of Aging." 21 (2010): 853–65.

"Prevention of Alzheimer's Disease: A Global Challenge for Next Generation Neuroscientists." 42 (2014): 515–23.

"Prevention of Alzheimer's Disease: Moving Backward through the Lifespan." 33 (2013): 465–69.

"A Review of the Major Vascular Risk Factors Related to Alzheimer's Disease." 32 (2012): 521–30.

"Targets for the Prevention of Dementia." 20 (2010): 915–24.

"Vascular Risk Factors: Imaging and Neuropathologic Correlates." 20 (2010): 699–709.

Journal of Biological Chemistry
"Apolipoprotein E Promotes β-Amyloid Trafficking and Degradation by Modulating Microglial Cholesterol Levels." 287 (2012): 2032–44.

Journal of Clinical and Experimental Neuropsychology
"Vascular and Cognitive Functions Associated with Cardiovascular Disease in the Elderly." 31 (2009): 96–110.

Journal of Gerontology: Series A, Biological Sciences and Medical Sciences
"Plasma HDL Levels Highly Correlate with Cognitive Function in Exceptional Longevity." 57 (2002): 712–15.

Journal of Internal Medicine
"Advances in the Prevention of Alzheimer's Disease and Dementia." 275 (2014): 229–50.

Journal of Neurology, Neurosurgery, and Psychiatry
"Cognitive Decline Precedes Late-Life Longitudinal Changes in Vascular Risk Factors." 81 (2010): 1028–32.

"Statins Are Associated with a Reduced Risk of Alzheimer Disease Regardless of Lipophilicity: The Rotterdam Study." 80 (2009): 13–17.

Journal of Nutrition

"A Healthy Dietary Pattern at Midlife Is Associated with Subsequent Cognitive Performance." 142 (2012): 909–15.

"Long-Term Adherence to the Mediterranean Diet Is Associated with Overall Cognitive Status, but Not Cognitive Decline, in Women." 143 (2013): 493–99.

"(n-6) and (n-3) Polyunsaturated Fatty Acids and the Aging Brain: Food for Thought." 138 (2008): 2521–22.

Journal of Nutrition, Health, and Aging

"Paths to Alzheimer's Disease Prevention: From Modifiable Risk Factors to Biomarker Enrichment Strategies." 19 (2015): 154–63.

Journal of the American College of Cardiology

"Improving Global Vascular Risk Prediction with Behavioral and Anthropometric Factors: The Multiethnic NOMAS (Northern Manhattan Cohort Study)." 54 (2009): 2303–11.

Journal of the American Geriatrics Society

"Coronary Artery Calcium: Associations with Brain Magnetic Resonance Imaging Abnormalities and Cognitive Status." 53 (2005): 609–15.

"Effect of Exercise on Cognitive Performance in Community-Dwelling Older Adults: Review of Intervention Trials and Recommendations for Public Health Practice and Research." 59 (2011): 704–16.

"Increases in Serum Non-High-Density Lipoprotein Cholesterol May Be Beneficial in Some High-Functioning Older Adults: MacArthur Studies of Successful Aging." 52 (2004): 487–94.

"A Longitudinal Study of Cardiorespiratory Fitness and Cognitive Function in Healthy Older Adults." 51 (2003): 459–65.

Journal of the American Heart Association

"The American Heart Association Life's Simple 7 and Incident Cognitive Impairment: The Reasons for Geographic and Racial Differences in Stroke (REGARDS) Study." 3 (2014): e000635.

"Effects of Daily Almond Consumption on Cardiometabolic Risk and Abdominal Adiposity in Healthy Adults with Elevated LDL Cholesterol: A Randomized Controlled Trial." 4 (2015): e000993.

"Impact of Nonoptimal Intakes of Saturated, Polyunsaturated, and Trans Fat on Global Burdens of Coronary Heart Disease." 5 (2016): e002891.

Journal of the American Medical Association

"Adherence to a Mediterranean Diet, Cognitive Decline, and Risk of Dementia." 302 (2009): 638–48.

"Brain Infarction and the Clinical Expression of Alzheimer Disease: The Nun Study." 277 (1997): 813–17.

"Effect of Physical Activity on Cognitive Function in Older Adults at Risk for Alzheimer Disease: A Randomized Trial." 300 (2008): 1027–37.

"Low-Density Lipoprotein Cholesterol and the Risk of Dementia with Stroke." 282 (1999): 254–60.

"Mixed Dementia: Emerging Concepts and Therapeutic Implications." 292 (2004): 2901–8.

"Physical Activity, Diet, and Risk of Alzheimer Disease." 302 (2009): 627–37.

"Physical Activity, Including Walking, and Cognitive Function in Older Women." 292 (2004): 1454–61.

Journal of the American Medical Association Neurology

"Association of Serum Docosahexaenoic Acid with Cerebral Amyloidosis." 73 (2016): 1208–16.

"Associations between Serum Cholesterol Levels and Cerebral Amyloidosis." 71 (2014): 195–200.

Journal of the Neurological Sciences

"Late and Early Onset Dementia: What Is the Role of Vascular Factors? A Retrospective Study." 322 (2012): 170–75.

"Neuropathological Evaluation of Mixed Dementia." 257 (2007): 80–87.

"Vascular Factors in Dementia: An Overview." 226 (2004): 19–23.

Lancet

"A Two-Year Multidomain Intervention of Diet, Exercise, Cognitive Training, and Vascular Risk Monitoring versus Control to Prevent Cognitive Decline in At-Risk Elderly People (FINGER): A Randomized Controlled Trial." 385 (2015): 2255–63.

"Vascular Dementia." 386 (2015): 1698–706.

Lancet Neurology

"The Age-Dependent Relation of Blood Pressure to Cognitive Function and Dementia." 4 (2005): 487–99.

"Leisure-Time Physical Activity at Midlife and the Risk of Dementia and Alzheimer's Disease." 4 (2005): 705–11.

"Potential for Primary Prevention of Alzheimer's Disease: An Analysis of Population-Based Data." 13 (2014): 788–94.

"The Projected Effect of Risk Factor Reduction on Alzheimer's Disease Prevalence." 10 (2011): 819–28.

"Risk Score for the Prediction of Dementia Risk in Twenty Years among Middle-Aged People: A Longitudinal, Population-Based Study." 5 (2006): 735–41.

Mayo Clinic Proceedings

"Physical Exercise as a Preventive or Disease-Modifying Treatment of Dementia and Brain Aging." 86 (2011): 876–84.

Medicine and Science in Sports and Exercise

"Associations between Physical Activity Dose and Health-Related Quality of Life." 36 (2004): 890–96.

Molecular Psychiatry

"Dietary Patterns and Cognitive Decline in an Australian Study of Aging." 20 (2015): 860–66.

National Weight Control Registry

"Long-Term Weight Loss Maintenance." 82 (2005): 222S–225S.

Nature Clinical Practice: Neurology

"Fish Consumption, Long-Chain Omega-3 Fatty Acids and Risk of Cognitive Decline or Alzheimer Disease: A Complex Association." 5 (2009): 140–52.

"Vascular Cognitive Impairment." 2 (2006): 538–47.

Nature Reviews: Neurology

"Changing Perspectives Regarding Late-Life Dementia." 5 (2009): 649–58.

Neurobiology of Aging

"Contribution of Vascular Pathology to the Clinical Expression of Dementia." 31 (2010): 1710–20.

"Coronary Risk Correlates with Cerebral Amyloid Deposition." 33 (2012): 1979–87.

"Linking Cerebrovascular Defense Mechanisms in Brain Aging and Alzheimer's Disease." 30 (2009): 1512–14.

"Serum Total Cholesterol, Statins, and Cognition in Non-demented Elderly." 30 (2009): 1006–9.

"Vascular Risk Factors for Alzheimer's Disease: An Epidemiologic Perspective." 21 (2000): 153–60.

Neuroepidemiology

"Risk Factors for Dementia in the Cardiovascular Health Cognition Study." 22 (2003): 13–22.

NeuroImage

"Combined Omega-3 Fatty Acids, Aerobic Exercise, and Cognitive Stimulation Prevents Decline in Gray Matter Volume of the Frontal, Parietal, and Cingulate Cortex in Patients with Mild Cognitive Impairment." 131 (2016): 226–38.

Neurology

"Aggregation of Vascular Risk Factors and Risk of Incident Alzheimer Disease." 65 (2005): 545–51.

"Association of Alzheimer Disease Pathology with Abnormal Lipid Metabolism: The Hisayama Study." 77 (2011): 1068–75.

"Associations of Vegetable and Fruit Consumption with Age-Related Cognitive Change." 67 (2006): 1370–76.

"Atherosclerosis and AD: Analysis of Data from the US National Alzheimer's Coordinating Center." 64 (2005): 494–500.

"Being Physically Active May Protect the Brain from Alzheimer Disease." 78 (2012): 1290–91.

"Blood-Brain Barrier Impairment in Alzheimer's Disease: Stability and Functional Significance." 68 (2007): 1809–14.

"Cardiovascular Risk Factors and Cognitive Decline in Middle-Aged Adults." 56 (2001): 42–48.

"Cerebral Infarcts in Patients with Autopsy-Proven Alzheimer's Disease: CERAD, Part XVIII. Consortium to Establish a Registry for Alzheimer's Disease." 51 (1998): 159–62.

"Clinical Trial Efforts in Alzheimer Disease: Why Test Statins?" 74 (2010): 945–46.

"Clinico-Pathologic Studies in Dementia: Nondemented Subjects with Pathologically Confirmed Alzheimer's Disease." 38 (1988): 1682–87.

"Dietary Fat Intake and Six-Year Cognitive Change in an Older Biracial Community Population." 62 (2004): 1573–79.

"Dietary Intake of Fatty Acids and Fish in Relation to Cognitive Performance at Middle Age." 62 (2004): 275–80.

"Executive Function, but Not Memory, Associates with Incident Coronary Heart Disease and Stroke." 85 (2015): 783–89.

"Impact of Plasma Lipids and Time on Memory Performance in Healthy Elderly without Dementia." 64 (2005): 1378–83.

"Incidence and Risk Factors of Vascular Dementia and Alzheimer's Disease in a Defined Elderly Japanese Population: The Hisayama Study." 45 (1995): 1161–68.

"Mediterranean Diet and Alzheimer Disease Mortality." 69 (2007): 1084–93.

"Mediterranean Diet and Brain Structure in a Multiethnic Elderly Cohort." 85 (2015): 1744–51.

"Midlife Cardiovascular Risk Factors and Risk of Dementia in Late Life." 64 (2005): 277–81.

"Midlife Vascular Risk Factor Exposure Accelerates Structural Brain Aging and Cognitive Decline." 77 (2011): 461–68.

"Midlife Vascular Risk Factors and Late-Life Mild Cognitive Impairment: A Population-Based Study." 56 (2001): 1683–89.

"Mixed Brain Pathologies Account for Most Dementia Cases in Community-Dwelling Older Persons." 69 (2007): 2197–204.

"Physical Activity and Dementia Risk in the Elderly: Findings from a Prospective Italian Study." 70 (2008): 1786–94.

"Physical Activity Predicts Gray Matter Volume in Late Adulthood: The Cardiovascular Health Study." 75 (2010): 1415–22.

"Predicting Risk of Dementia in Older Adults: The Late-Life Dementia Risk Index." 73 (2009): 173–79.

"Relation of DASH- and Mediterranean-like Dietary Patterns to Cognitive Decline in Older Persons." 83 (2014): 1410–16.

"Statins and Cognitive Function in the Elderly: The Cardiovascular Health Study." 65 (2005): 1388–94.

"Statins, Incident Alzheimer Disease, Change in Cognitive Function, and Neuropathology." 70 (2008): 1795–802.

"Total Daily Physical Activity and the Risk of AD and Cognitive Decline in Older Adults." 78 (2012): 1323–29.

"Treatment of Vascular Risk Factors Is Associated with Slower Decline in Alzheimer Disease." 73 (2009): 674–80.

"Vascular Risk Factors and Cognitive Impairment in a Stroke-Free Cohort." 77 (2011): 1729–36.

"Vascular Risk Factors and Dementia: How to Move Forward?" 72 (2009): 368–74.

"Vascular Risk Factors, Incidence of MCI, and Rates of Progression to Dementia." 63 (2004): 1882–91.

"Vascular Risk Factors Promote Conversion from Mild Cognitive Impairment to Alzheimer Disease." 76 (2011): 1485–91.

New England Journal of Medicine

"Explaining the Decrease in U.S. Deaths from Coronary Disease, 1980–2000." 356 (2007): 2388–98.

"Incidence of Dementia over Three Decades in the Framingham Heart Study." 374 (2016): 523–32.

"Primary Prevention of Cardiovascular Disease with a Mediterranean Diet." 368 (2013): 1279–90.

"Silent Brain Infarcts and the Risk of Dementia and Cognitive Decline." 348 (2003): 1215–22.

Nutrition Reviews

"Scientific Evidence of Interventions Using the Mediterranean Diet: A Systematic Review." 64 (2006): 27–47.

Obesity

"Midlife Obesity and Dementia: Meta-analysis and Adjusted Forecast of Dementia Prevalence in the United States and China." 21 (2013): 51–55.

Obesity Reviews

"Body Mass Index in Midlife and Late-Life as a Risk Factor for Dementia: A Meta-analysis of Prospective Studies." 12 (2011): 426–37.

"Obesity and Central Obesity as Risk Factors for Incident Dementia and Its Subtypes: A Systematic Review and Meta-analysis." 9 (2008): 204–18.

Plos One

"Changes in Cognition and Mortality in Relation to Exercise in Late Life: A Population Based Study." 3 (2008): 3124.

Public Health Nutrition

"n-3 Fatty Acids, Hypertension, and Risk of Cognitive Decline among Older Adults in the Atherosclerosis Risk in Communities (ARIC) Study." 11 (2008): 17–29.

Stroke

"Carotid Intimal Medial Thickness Predicts Cognitive Decline among Adults without Clinical Vascular Disease." 40 (2009): 3180–85.

"Increasing Rates of Dementia at Time of Declining Mortality from Stroke." 37 (2006): 1155–59.

"The Lifetime Risk of Stroke: Estimates from the Framingham Study." 37 (2006): 345–50.

"Progression of Cerebral Small Vessel Disease in Relation to Risk Factors and Cognitive Consequences: Rotterdam Scan Study." 39 (2008): 2712–19.

"Reducing the Risk of Dementia: Efficacy of Long-Term Treatment of Hypertension." 37 (2006): 1165–70.

"Vascular Contributions to Cognitive Impairment and Dementia: A Statement for Healthcare Professionals from the American Heart Association/American Stroke Association." 42 (2011): 2672–713.

Trends in Neurosciences

"Neurovascular Mechanisms of Alzheimer's Neurodegeneration." 28 (2005): 202–8.

University of Kuopio, Finland

"Midlife Serum Cholesterol and Increased Risk of Alzheimer's and Vascular Dementia Three Decades Later." 28 (2009): 75–80.

Vascular Health and Risk Management

"Vascular Risk Factors, Cognitive Decline, and Dementia." 4 (2008): 363–81.

Zeitschrift für Gerontologie und Geriatrie

"A Brief Update on Dementia Prevention." 45 (2012): 7–10.

Other Sources

National Institute on Aging. "The Search for Alzheimer's Prevention Strategies." National Institutes of Health. US Department of Health and Human Services. September 1, 2012. https://www.nia.nih.gov/alz heimers/publication/preventing-alzheimers-disease/search-alzheimers -prevention-strategies.

Prince, M., E. Albanese, M. Guerchet, and M. Prina. World Alzheimer Report 2014. "Dementia and Risk Reduction: An Analysis of Protective and Modifiable Risk Factors." London: Alzheimer's Disease International.

UK Health Prevention First Forum. January 30, 2014. "Promoting Brain Health: Developing a Prevention Agenda Linking Dementia and Noncommunicable Diseases." St. Brides Foundation, Blackfriars, London.

Richard Furman, MD, FACS, spent over thirty years as a vascular surgeon. Furman is past president of the North Carolina chapter of the American College of Surgeons, past president of the North Carolina Surgical Society, and a two-term governor of the American College of Surgeons. He is cofounder of World Medical Mission, the medical arm of Samaritan's Purse, and a member of the board of Samaritan's Purse. He lives in Boone, North Carolina.

For more information, please visit www.RichardFurman.com.

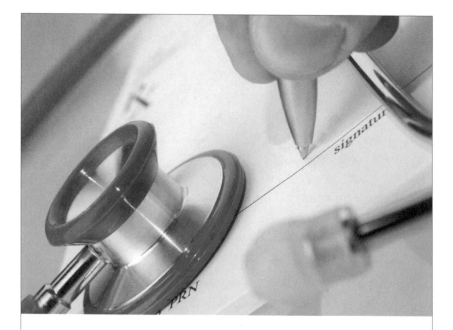

Visit
RICHARDFURMAN.COM
for further reading and information.

♦ ♦ ♦

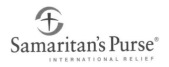

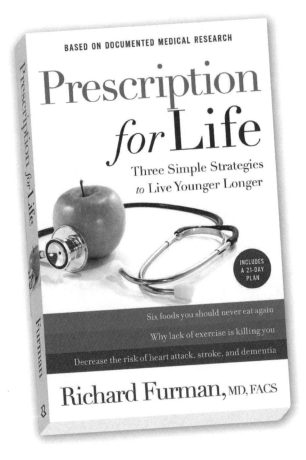
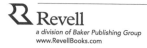

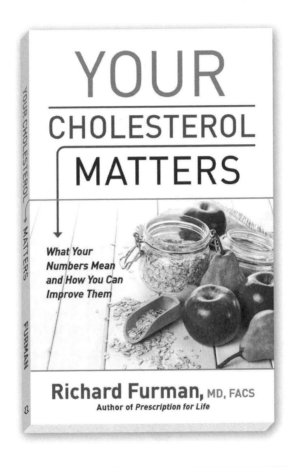

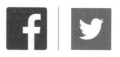
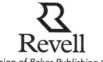